Anti-Inflammatory-Chicken

To Heal Your Immune System And Fight Immation

Richard V. Jowett

Contents

Chapter One

INTRODUCTION

Anti-Inflammatory-Chicken-Cookbook

To Heal Your Immune System And Fight Immation, Try These Chicken Recipes, Sides, And Sauces

Author : Richard V. Jowett

Chapter Two

VEGETABLE-FILLED SOLE

Preparation time: 10 minutes Cooking Time: 15 minutes Serving Size: 4\sIngredients:

12 c. vegetable broth, split 1 carrot, finely sliced and divided zucchini, thinly sliced and split 2 shallots, sliced and thinly split tbsp. snipped fresh chives 4 tsp extra-virgin olive oil, split

sole fillets, 5 oz. black peppercorns, ground slices of lemon

Salt

Directions:

Preheat the oven to 4250 degrees Fahrenheit.

Cut the aluminum foil into pieces of a reasonable size.

Place a fillet on one side of the aluminum foil and season with salt and pepper.

On top of the fillet, layer shallots, zucchini, and 14 carrots each. 12 teaspoon chives drizzled on top

2 tablespoons broth, 1 tablespoon olive oil over the fish and veggies

Seal the package and place it on a large baking sheet.

Make additional packets by repeating the process with the remaining components.

Bake the packets for fifteen minutes on the sheet in a preheated oven.

Remove the foil and transfer the contents, together with the liquid, to a serving platter.

Serve with lemon wedges for garnish.

Information about nutrition: Protein: 9.94 g Fat: 7.96 g Carbohydrates: 4.92 g Calories: 130 kcal Protein: 9.94 g Fat: 7.96 g Carbohydrates: 4.92 g

SALMON BOWLS WITH SOUVLAKI SPICES

Preparation time: 10 minutes Cooking Time: 20 minutes Serving Size: 4 components:

For the salmon, prepare the following:

14 cup extra virgin olive oil

14 teaspoon black pepper, freshly ground

a quarter teaspoon of salt

1 tblsp balsamic vinaigrette 1 tablespoon garlic, minced

1 tablespoon sweet paprika, smoked 2 tblsp. fresh oregano, chopped 4 salmon fillets (4 oz.) 1 lemon's juice

To make the bowls:

12 cup Kalamata olives, sliced

a quarter-cup of sour cream

1 large sliced tomato 1 diced cucumber

1 red bell pepper, peeled and sliced into strips

1 thinly sliced yellow bell pepper

1 zucchini, sliced lengthwise into 12-inch strips 2 tblsp. extra virgin olive oil

6 oz. crumbled feta cheese

Directions:

To create the salmon, follow these steps:

Prepare the fish by marinating it. Combine the olive oil, lemon juice, oregano, garlic, vinegar, paprika, salt, and pepper in a medium-sized container. Place the fish in the marinade and flip it to coat it completely. Allow the salmon to marinate for 15 to 20 minutes in the covered container.

Cook the fish on the grill. Preheat the grill to medium-high heat and cook the fish for four to five minutes each side, or until just cooked through. Place the fish on a platter and set it away.

Grill the veggies for the bowls. Combine the oil, red and yellow bell peppers, and zucchini in a medium-sized container. Grill the veggies for 3 minutes each side, turning once, until they are moderately browned and tender.

Before you serve, put everything together. Divide the grilled veggies into four serving dishes. Add cucumber, tomato, olives, feta cheese, and sour cream to each container. Serve immediately by placing 1 salmon fillet on top of each container.

Information about nutrition: 553 calories 44g total fat Carbohydrates in total: 10g Sodium: 531mg; Fiber: 3g; Net carbs: 7g 30 g protein

NOODLES WITH SUPER SESAME CHICKEN

Preparation time: 10 minutes Cooking time: 10 minutes Serving Size: 12 cup of 12 cup of 12 cup of 12 cup of 12 cup of 12 cup of 12 cup of 12 cup of 12 cup of Snap peas (sugar)

12 oz. orange juice

1 sliced carrot

1 cup Japanese Udon (rice/buckwheat noodles) 1 tsp. ginger, chopped into a thumb size piece 2 tsp. sesame seed free-range

skinless chicken breasts Coconut Oil is a kind of vegetable oil that is

Directions:

In a frying pan, heat 1 tsp oil over medium heat.

Cook the chopped chicken breast for about ten to fifteen minutes, or until fully done.

Put the noodles, carrots, and peas in a saucepan of boiling water for about five minutes while the chicken is cooking. Drain.

To create the dressing, put the ginger, sesame seeds, 1 tsp oil, and orange juice in a jar.

Toss the chicken, noodles, carrots, and peas with the dressing after the chicken and noodles are cooked and drained.

Warm or cooled is fine.

Information about nutrition: 168 calories per serving; 5.31 grams of protein; 8.66 grams of fat 19.34 g carbohydrate

CABBAGE WITH RED CABBAGE AND CHEESE

Preparation time: 5 minutes Cooking time: 12 minutes Serving Size: 4\sIngredients:

1 tbsp. extra virgin olive oil and 14 cup extra virgin olive oil

14 tsp freshly ground black pepper

14 teaspoon salt

1 pound walnuts

1 tbsp. blue cheese crumbles 1 tablespoon Dijon mustard, 1 tablespoon butter, thinly sliced scallions, 1 tablespoon pure maple syrup red wine vinegar, 3 tbsp.

8 cups finely sliced red cabbage

Directions:

To make the vinaigrette, combine all of the ingredients in a mixing bowl.

1. In a food processor or blender, combine the blue cheese, 14 cup olive oil, mustard, vinegar, salt, and pepper until the mixture has a creamy consistency.

To make the salad:

Place a piece of parchment paper next to the burner.

In a medium-sized frying pan, heat 1 tablespoon of oil over medium heat and add the walnuts, cooking for about 2 minutes.

Now season with salt and pepper, drizzle with maple syrup, and simmer for three to five minutes, turning occasionally, until the nuts are evenly coated.

Transfer to the paper and use a spoon to pour the remaining syrup over them. Cool for about five minutes after separating the nuts.

Place the cabbage and scallions in a large container and mix with the vinaigrette. As toppers, add the walnuts and blue cheese.

Information about nutrition: 232 calories 19 gram of fat saturating 4 gram of fat Sodium (g): 267 g

Carbohydrates: 12 g 2 gram sugar fiber 8 milligram 5 gram sugar added 4 gram protein PISTACHIOS AND RICE

Preparation time: 10 minutes Cooking time: 20 minutes Serving Size: 6\sIngredients:

14 cup pistachios, raw (or more for decoration)

12 cup dill leaves, chopped and packed

12 tsp turmeric powder

12 CUP BASMATRIC RICE (rinsed in a colander and soaked in water for approximately 30 minutes, or more)

1 teaspoon of extra virgin olive oil 1 medium onion, thinly sliced 2 baby leaves, dried

3 c. vegetable stock (or 3 c. water)

5 green cardamom pods, gently smashed black peppercorns, ground (to taste)

season with salt to taste

Directions:

Warm the oil in a large deep skillet and add the cardamom. Heat it for about 1 minute, or until it acquires a light brown color, then add the onion. Cook for 1-2 minutes over medium-high heat.

Combine the dill leaves, turmeric, and pistachios in a mixing bowl. After that, add the rice and stir-fry for about a minute.

Combine the vegetable stock, black pepper, and salt to taste in a large mixing bowl and bring to a boil.

Cook for around fifteen minutes on low to moderate heat with the lid on the pan.

Remove it from the heat and let the rice aside (covered) for about ten minutes. Then fluff it with a fork and garnish with additional pistachios if desired.

Enjoy!

Calories: 90 kcal; Protein: 3.36 g; Fat: 5.08 g; Calories: 90 kcal; Calories: 90 kcal; Calories: 90 kcal; Calories: 90 kcal; Calories: 90 kcal; Cal 8.39 g carbohydrate

CARROTS ROASTED

Preparation time: 10 minutes Cooking time: 40 minutes Serving Size: 4\sIngredients:

14 teaspoon pepper, ground

12 tsp rosemary (chopped)

a quarter teaspoon of salt

1 peeled and sliced onion teaspoon chopped thyme tablespoons extra-virgin olive oil 8 peeled and sliced carrots
Directions:

Preheat oven to 425 degrees Fahrenheit.

Toss the onions and carrots with rosemary, thyme, pepper, and salt in a container. Place on a baking sheet.

Cook for 40 minutes at 350°F. Browning and softening onions and carrots are required.

Calories: 126; Carbohydrates: 16g; Protein: 2g 6 g total fat; 2 g protein 4 g of fiber

8 g of sugar 286 mg sodium

CAULIFLOWER WITH CURRIED ROAST

Preparation time: 5 minutes Cooking time: 30 minutes Serving Size: 4\sIngredients:

a quarter teaspoon of salt

1 and a half tablespoons of extra virgin olive oil

1 cauliflower head, sliced into florets 1 teaspoon seeds of cumin

curry powder (1 teaspoon) mustard seeds (1 teaspoon)

Directions:

Preheat the oven to 375°F (190°C).

Using cooking spray, grease a baking pan.

Place all ingredients in a jar.

Toss well to coat.

Place the veggie on a baking pan and bake it.

30 minutes of roasting

Serve and have fun!

Nutritional Information: 67 calories, 6 grams of fat, 4 grams of carbohydrates, and 2 grams of protein

PARSNIPS ROASTED TIME TO PREPARE: 5 MINUTES Cooking time: 30 minutes Serving Size: 4\sIngredients:

1 tbsp extra-virgin extra-virgin olive oil 1 teaspoon salt (kosher)

12 teaspoon seasoning (Italian) 2 pound parsnips

Parsley, chopped for decorating

Directions:

Preheat oven to 400 degrees Fahrenheit.

Parsnips should be peeled. Make one-inch slices out of them.

In a jar, combine the seasoning, salt, and oil.

This should be spread out on your baking sheet. It has to be in one layer.

Roast for 30 minutes. Every 10 minutes, give it a good stir.

Transfer to a plate. Use parsley as a finishing touch.

Calories 124; Carbohydrates 20; Total Fat 4; Protein 2; Fiber 4; Sugar 5; Calories 124; Carbohydrates 20; Total Fat 4; Protein 2; Fiber 4; Sugar 5; Calories 124; Calories 124; Calories 124; Calories 124; Calories 124; Calories 124; Calories 124; Calories 124 Sodium (mg): 550

SOUVLAKI WITH CIPOLLINI AND BELL PEPPER CHICKEN

Preparation time: 5 minutes Cooking time: 12 minutes Serving Size: 2-4\sIngredients:

red bell pepper, chopped into bits 12 cup lemon juice 1 tsp rosemary leaves for garnish 2 cubed chicken breasts, minced garlic cloves 2 tbsp. extra virgin olive oil

2–4 lemon wedges for garnish Small cipollini, 8 oz.

Season with salt and black pepper to taste.

Directions:

Save the skewers with the chicken, bell pepper, and cipollini for later. Place the chicken skewers in a container with half of the oil, garlic, salt, black pepper, and lemon juice. Cover the jar and place it in the fridge for at least 2 hours to marinate the chicken.

Preheat the grill to high and cook the skewers for about six minutes on each side. Remove the rosemary leaves and lemon wedges before serving.

Calories: 363; Fat: 14.2g Net; Carbs: 4.2g; Protein: 32.5g

CHICKEN WITH COCONUT, CURRY, AND CASHEE

Preparation time: 15 minutes Cooking time: 7–8 hours Serving Size: 4 components:

12 cup white onion, diced

12 teaspoon sugar (coconut)

12 teaspoon black pepper, freshly ground 1 full-fat coconut milk can (14 oz.)

1 tablespoon curry paste (red) 1 teaspoon powdered garlic

1 teaspoon salt

12 cup cashews, unsalted

112 cup Bone Broth for Chicken pound boneless, skinless chicken breasts

Directions:

Combine broth, coconut milk, garlic powder, red curry paste, salt, pepper, and coconut sugar in a container. Stir everything together completely.

In a slow cooker, combine the chicken, cashews, and onion. On top of it, pour the coconut milk mixture.

Set your cooker on low and secure the lid. Cook for eight hours, or until the internal temperature of the chicken reaches 165°F and the juices flow clear when tested with a meat thermometer.

Using a fork, shred the chicken and combine it with the cooking liquid. Remove the chicken from the soup and chop it into bite-size pieces with a knife before returning it to the slow cooker and serving.

Information about nutrition: calorie count: 714 43 g total fat Carbohydrates (total): 21g Sugar (total): 5g 3 g of fiber 57 g protein 1,606mg sodium

GREENS & CREAMY CHICKEN

Preparation time: 10 minutes Cooking Time: 20 minutes Serving Size: 4\sIngredients:

1 cup of liquid 1 cup chicken stock Cream\slb. 1 tsp. skins on chicken thighs Cups of Italian herbs Leafy greens with a dark color 2 tablespoons 2 tbsp coconut flour 2 tbsp coconut oil butter that has been melted

Salt & Pepper (your preference)

Directions:

Using the medium-high temperature setting on the stovetop, pour oil into a frying pan.

Remove the chicken's bones and season with salt and pepper. Cook the chicken until it is fully cooked.

To make the sauce, melt the butter in a large saucepan. To form a thick paste, whisk in the flour. Whisk in the cream gradually. Once the water has to a boil, add the herbs.

Place the chicken on the counter and pour the stock over it.

Whisk the cream sauce while deglazing the pan. Add the greens and toss them in the sauce until they are well coated.

Before serving, place the thighs on the greens to warm up.

Information about nutrition: calorie count: 446 Net 3 g of carbohydrates Fat in total: 38 g (about) 18 g protein

LETTUCE WRAPS WITH CURRY CHICKEN

Preparation time: 15 minutes

Cooking time: 10 minutes

Serving Size: 5

Ingredients:\s.

25 oz. onion, minced 1 pound of riced cauliflower Skinless and boneless chicken thighs 1 teaspoon of black pepper

garlic cloves, minced 2 tablespoons 2 tsp. ghee Curry powder is a spice used in cooking. Lettuce leaves, 5-6

Sour cream that is keto-friendly (as you wish - count the carbs) season with salt to taste

Directions:

Garlic and onions should be minced. Place on the side to be used later.

Remove the chicken's bones and skin, then cut it into one-inch pieces.

Melt 2 tablespoons ghee in a frying skillet on the heat. Add the onion and cook until it is golden. Combine the chicken, garlic, pepper, and salt in a mixing bowl.

Cook for a further 8 minutes. Combine the remaining ghee, riced cauliflower, and curry in a mixing bowl. Stir until everything is well blended.

Prepare the lettuce leaves and toss them in with the other ingredients.

Serve with a dollop of sour cream on top.

Information about nutrition: Net calories: 554 7 g of carbohydrates 36 g total fat content; 50 g protein content

YUM YUM YUM YUM YUM YUM YUM YUM YUM

Preparation time: 10 minutes

Cooking time: 4 hours and 50 minutes

Serving Size: 4\sIngredients:

14 cup chopped parsley 1 sliced celery stalk 1 duck, medium bay leaves (two)

2 tablespoons dried thyme 8 garlic cloves, minced 2 yellow onions, diced

a sprinkle of black pepper and a pinch of salt a teaspoon of Provence herbs

To make the sauce, combine the following ingredients.

14 teaspoon Provence herbs

12 CUP WINE (WHITE)

sugar (12 teaspoon)

1 and 12 cup pitted and chopped black olives 1 quart chicken broth 1 tablespoon paste de tomate 1 chopped yellow onion 3 quarts liquid

Directions:

Place thyme, parsley, garlic, and 2 onions in a baking dish.

Place the duck in the pan and season with salt, pepper, and 1 teaspoon herbs de Provence.

Preheat the oven to 475°F and roast for around 10 minutes.

Cover the dish, lower the heat to 275°F, and roast the duck for three hours and thirty minutes.

Meanwhile, heat a skillet over medium heat, add 1 yellow onion, stir, and cook for 10 minutes.

Cover, reduce the heat to low, and simmer for an hour with tomato paste, stock, sugar, 14 teaspoon herbs de Provence, olives, and water.

Carve the duck on a work surface, discard the bones, and divide across plates.

Serve immediately after sprinkling the sauce all over.

Information about nutrition: 254 calories, 3 grams of fat 3 g fiber 8 g carbohydrate 13 grams of protein

UNDER PRESSURE DELIGHTFUL TERIYAKI CHICKEN

Preparation time: 5 minutes Cooking Time: 20 minutes Serving Size: 14 cup apple cider vinegar 34 cup brown sugar 8 ingredients

a third of a cup of low-sodium soy sauce 1 tsp chicken broth 1 cup chicken broth a tbsp. of pepper and a tbsp. of garlic powder 2 tbsp. ginger powder

20 oz. crushed canned pineapple

3 kilos Chicken Thighs, Boneless and Skinless

Directions: Combine all of the ingredients, except the chicken, in a mixing bowl. Place the chicken meat in the pan and toss to coat.

Secure the cover, press POULTRY, and cook on High for approximately 20 minutes. Turn the valve to the "open" position for a rapid pressure release.

Information about nutrition: 352 calories Carbohydrates: 31g Fat: 11g 31 g protein

DOUBLE CHEESE CHEESE CHEESE CHEESE CHE CHICKEN IN ITALY

Preparation time: 10 minutes Cooking Time: 20 minutes Serving Size: 2\s

Ingredients:

12 CUP CREAM CREAM CREAM CREAM CREAM C

1 cup grated Asiago cheese 1 tsp Italian spice blend 2 cups baby spinach 2 chicken drumsticks

Directions:

1 tbsp. oil, heated over moderate to high heat in a deep frying pan Reserve the chicken drumsticks after searing them for seven to eight minutes, or until nicely browned on both sides.

Pour in 12 cup chicken bone broth, then add the spinach and simmer for another five minutes, or until the spinach has wilted.

Cook for 5 minutes further after adding the Italian spice blend, cream cheese, Asiago cheese, and the reserved chicken drumsticks. Warm the dish before serving.

Information about nutrition: 589 Calories: 46g Fat: 5.8g Carbohydrates: 37.5g 2 g protein Fiber

MIX OF DUCK BREAST AND BLACKBERRIES

Preparation time: 10 minutes Cooking time: twenty-five minutes 4 servings (about)

14 cup chicken stock, 1 teaspoon thyme, 1 teaspoon thyme, 1 teaspoon thyme 12 cup water, a spoonful of butter, and a tablespoon of balsamic vinegar 2 tablespoons sugar duck breasts 2 teaspoons cornflour

blackberries, 4 oz.

Season with salt and black pepper to taste.

Directions:

Using paper towels, pat dry the duck breasts. Set aside for half an hour after scoring the skin and seasoning it with salt and pepper to taste.

Cook for eight minutes with the breasts skin side down in a pan over medium heat.

Cook for another half-minute after flipping the breasts.

Place the duck breasts skin side up in a baking dish and bake for fifteen minutes at 425 degrees F.

Remove the meat from the oven and set it aside to cool for ten minutes before cutting it.

Meanwhile, put the sugar in a skillet and melt it over medium heat, stirring constantly.

Remove the pan from the heat and add the blackberries, water, stock, and balsamic vinegar.

Heat this mixture over a low heat and simmer until the sauce has been reduced by half.

Transfer the sauce to a new pan, stir in the cornflour and water, heat again, and simmer for four minutes, or until it thickens.

Add the salt and pepper, as well as the butter, and stir well. Cut the duck breasts in halves, divide into plates, and top with the berry sauce.

Information about nutrition: calorie count: 320 fifteen pounds of fat fifteen grams of fiber 16 g carbohydrate 11 grams of protein

Chapter Three

SALAD WITH DUCK BREASTS

Preparation time: 10 minutes Cooking Time: 20 minutes Serving Size: 4\sIngredients:

1 frisee head, torn

a quarter-cup of lemon juice

1 teaspoon grated lemon zest duck breasts, boneless but with skin on, sliced into 4 pieces 1 teaspoon orange zest, grated 2 orange segments, peeled and sliced

2 small heads of lettuce, cleaned and cut into little pieces 2 tablespoons chopped chives 2 teaspoons sugar 2 tablespoons minced shallot

white wine vinegar, 3 tblsp. Season with salt and black pepper to taste. 1 tblsp. canola oil

Directions:

Warm a small deep frying pan over moderate to high heat, then add the vinegar and sugar, stir to combine, and cook for five minutes, then remove from the heat.

Stir in the orange zest, lemon zest, and lemon juice before setting aside for a few minutes.

Mix in the shallot, salt, and pepper to taste, as well as the oil, and set aside.

Dry the duck pieces, score the skin, remove the excess fat, and season with salt and pepper.

Warm a pan over medium to high heat for a minute, then place duck breast pieces skin side down in the pan and brown for eight minutes. Reduce the heat to moderate and cook for another four minutes.

Cook for three minutes on the other side, then transfer to a cutting board and cover with foil.

Combine the frisee and lettuce in a container, toss to combine, and divide among plates.

Slice the duck and place it on top, then add the orange segments, chives, and vinaigrette.

Information about nutrition: 320 calories, 4 grams of fat, and 4 grams of fiber 6 g carbohydrate 14 grams of protein

APRICOT SAUCE FOR DUCK BREAST

Preparation time: 10 minutes Cooking Time: 20 minutes Serving Size: 14 teaspoon cinnamon (ground), 14 teaspoon coriander (ground), 34 cup blackberries apricots, chopped cup apricots, chopped apricots, chopped apricots, chopped apricots,

2 teaspoons chopped red onions apple cider vinegar, 3 tblsp. 3 tablespoons chives, diced duck breasts, boneless apricot preserving teaspoons a smidgeon of olive oil

Season with salt and black pepper to taste.

Directions:

Season duck breasts with salt, pepper, coriander, and cinnamon, then place them on a hot grill pan over moderate to high heat and cook for a few minutes before flipping and cooking for another three minutes.

Return the duck breasts to the pan, add 3 tablespoons apricot preserves, heat for a minute, transfer to a cutting board, set aside for at least two minutes before slicing.

Put vinegar, onion, 2 tablespoons apricot preServings, apricots, blackberries, and chives in a skillet over medium heat, mix, and simmer for approximately three minutes.

Serve the sliced duck breasts on plates with apricot sauce drizzled on top.

Information about nutrition: Calories consumed: 275 4 g of fat 4 g fiber 7 g carbohydrate 12 g protein

SAUCE WITH DUCK LEGS AND WINE

Preparation time: 10 minutes

Cooking time: 1 hour and 30 minutes

Serving Size: 4\sIngredients:

12 cup stock (chicken)

1 and a half a gallon of red wine 1 sliced carrot

1 tblsp balsamic vinaigrette 1 teaspoon extra virgin olive oil

a teaspoon of dried rosemary 2 teaspoons sugar 2 shallots, chopped

2 tablespoons paste de tomate 4 trimmed duck legs black pepper with salt

Directions:

Warm the oil in a pan over medium to high heat.

Place the duck legs in the pan, season with salt and pepper, and cook for five minutes on both sides before transferring to a platter.

Place the shallots and carrots in the same pan over medium heat, stir, and cook for a few minutes.

Stir in the wine, tomato paste, stock, sugar, vinegar, and rosemary, then reduce to a low heat and cook for five minutes.

Return the duck legs, toss, and simmer for an hour and 30 minutes on low heat, stirring often. Divide the mixture amongst plates before serving.

Information about nutrition: Calories: 257 kcal / 14 kcal / 14 kcal / 14 kcal / 14 kcal Carbohydrates: 14 Fiber: 6 8 g protein

OLLA TAPADA DUCK STEW

Preparation time: 15 minutes Cooking time: 30 minutes Serving Size: 3\sIngredients:

12 cup peeled and cubed chayote

1 pound boneless, skinless duck breasts, cut into small bits 1 deveined and chopped red bell pepper

1 chopped shallot

1 teaspoon Mexican seasoning blend

2 teaspoons canola oil, heated in a clay pot over a moderate to high burner. Sauté the peppers and shallot for four minutes, or until tender.

Add the other ingredients, as well as 12 cups of water or chicken bone broth. Reduce the heat to medium-low until the mixture starts to boil.

Allow it to cook for eighteen to 22 minutes, partially covered, until well done. Enjoy!

Information about nutrition: 228 calories 9.5 grams fat 3.3 grams Carbohydrates: 30.6g Protein: 1g Fiber

TACOS WITH EASY CHICKEN

Preparation time: 5 minutes Cooking time: 2 minutes and 7 seconds Serving Size: 4\sIngredients:

12 c. salsa

12 cup Mexican cheese mixture 1 garlic clove, minced

1 cup pureed tomatoes

1 tablespoon Mexican seasoning mix 1 pound ground chicken 2 bacon pieces, coarsely chopped shallots, peeled and finely chopped 2 tbsp. room temperature butter

Directions:

Butter should be melted in a deep frying pan over a fairly high temperature. Cook the shallots until they are tender and fragrant.

Then, for about five minutes, sauté the garlic, chicken, and bacon, turning frequently and crushing with a fork. Toss in the Mexican spice mix.

Fold in the tomato puree and salsa; continue to cook for another five to seven minutes on low to moderate heat; set aside.

Wax paper should be used to line a baking sheet. To form "taco shells," place 4 stacks of shredded cheese on the baking sheet and gently press them down with a broad spatula.

Preheat the oven to 365°F and bake for six to seven minutes, or until the chocolate has melted. Allow for a ten-minute cooling period after removing the taco shells.

Information about nutrition: Calories: 535 33.3 g 4.8 g fat 47.9 g carbs 1.9 g protein Fiber

PEAR AND ONION GOOSE EXQUISITE

Preparation time: 15 minutes Cooking Time: 20 minutes Serving Size: 8\sIngredients:

a quarter teaspoon of garlic powder

12 cup onions, sliced

12 teaspoon pepper

12 pound goose, cut into large chunks 1 tablespoon Butter\stsp Cayenne Pepper 2 quarts tbsp. chicken broth Balsamic Vinegar is a kind of vinegar that comes from Italy. 3 peeled and sliced pears

Directions:

On SAUTÉ, melt the butter. Place the geese in the pan and cook until golden brown on both sides. Transfer to a plate. Cook for a few minutes after adding the onions. Return the geese to the oven to finish cooking.

Place the other ingredients in the pot, stir well to combine, and cover. Set the timer to eighteen minutes at High Pressure in the PRESSURE COOK/MANUAL mode. Make a fast release of pressure. Serve and have fun!

Information about nutrition: 313 calories Carbohydrates: 14 g 8 g of fat 38 g protein

HEALTHY GUMBO WITH TURKEY

Preparation time: 5 minutes

Cooking time: 2 hours Serving Size: 1 set of ingredients

12 cup of okra

1 tomato can (chopped) 1 quartered onion

1 tablespoon Olive oils that are extra virgin 1 turkey, whole

a few bay leaves

3 garlic cloves, chopped to taste black pepper Celery stalk, chopped In a stockpot, combine the first four ingredients with 2 cups of water and cook over high heat until boiling.

Reduce the heat to low and cook for approximately 50 minutes, or until the turkey is fully cooked.

Remove the turkey from the soup and drain it.

Heat the oil in a frying pan over medium heat and cook the remaining veggies for five to ten minutes.

Stir until the vegetables are mushy, then add to the broth.

Toss the tomatoes and turkey meat into the stock, stirring constantly.

Add the bay leaves and continue to simmer for another hour or until the sauce has thickened.

Enjoy it with a pinch of black pepper.

Information about nutrition: 261 calories, 11.72 grams of protein, 12.91 grams of fat, and 28.33 grams of carbohydrates

CHICKEN DRUMMIES FROM THE HIDDEN VALLEY

Preparation time: 15 minutes Cooking time: 30 minutes Serving Size: 4\sIngredients:

12 c. butter, melted

12 packets of chicken drumsticks Dry dressing mix from Hidden Valley 2 tblsp tbsp. hot sauce Vinegar Sticks of celery Paprika

Preheat the oven to 350 degrees Fahrenheit.

The chicken should be washed and dried.

Combine the dry dressing, melted butter, vinegar, and spicy sauce in a container. Stir until everything is well blended.

Place the drumsticks in a large plastic baggie and pour the sauce on top. Massage the sauce into the drumsticks until they are completely covered.

Place the chicken in a baking dish in a single layer. Paprika should be drizzled on top.

Preheat oven to 350°F and bake for 30 minutes, flipping halfway through.

Serve with crudités or a salad.

Calories: 155 calories; fat: 18 grams; carbohydrates: 96 grams; protein: 15 grams; sugars: 0.7 grams; sodium: 340 milligrams

CHICKEN KEBAB IN THE STYLE OF HOME

Preparation time: 10 minutes Cooking time: 10 minutes Serving Size: Ingredients for 2: 12 cup yogurt (Greek-style)

12 ounce Swiss cheese, chopped pound boneless, skinless, and halved chicken thighs 2 Roma tomatoes, chopped olive oil teaspoons

Directions:

In a glass storage container, combine the chicken thighs, yogurt, tomatoes, and olive oil. If you like, you may add mustard seeds, cinnamon, and sumac.

Cover and marinate for three to four hours in the refrigerator.

Make a thick log form out of the chicken thighs by threading them onto skewers. Grill the kebabs for three to four minutes on each side over medium to high heat.

Check the doneness of the meat with an instant-read thermometer; it should register about 165 degrees F.

Continue to simmer for another four minutes, or until the cheese has melted. Enjoy!

Information about nutrition: 498 Calories 23.2 g 6.2 g fat 61 g carbs 1.7 g protein Fiber

TAGINE WITH HONEY CHICKEN

Preparation Time: 60 minutes Cooking time: twenty-five minutes Serving Size: 12\sIngredients:

12 tsp. pepper, ground

12 teaspoon salt

34 tsp cinnamon powder 12 tablespoons honey

1 tbsp olive oil (extra virgin) 1 tablespoon fresh ginger, minced 1 tsp. coriander powder 1 tsp. cumin powder 1/8 teaspoon Cloves, ground

Kumquats, seeds and coarsely chopped, 12 oz. lbs. boneless, skinless chicken thighs 14-oz. vegetable broth 2 onions, thinly sliced

4 garlic cloves, slivered rinsed chickpeas (15 ounce)

Directions:

Preheat the oven to 3750 degrees Fahrenheit.

Heat the oil in a heatproof casserole over medium heat.

Add the onions and cook for approximately four minutes.

Add the garlic and ginger and cook for a minute.

Season with coriander, cumin, cloves, salt, pepper, and garlic cloves. 1 minute of sautéing

Add the kumquats, broth, chickpeas, and honey, then bring to a boil before removing from the heat.

Cover the dish and place it in the oven. Bake for fifteen minutes, stirring every fifteen minutes.

Serve and have fun!

Information about nutrition: Calories: 586 kcal, 15.5 g protein, 40.82 g fat 43.56 g carbohydrate

CHICKEN WITH A HONEY-MUSTARD LEMON MARINADE

Preparation time: 10 minutes Cooking Time: 20 minutes Serving Size: 4\sIngredients:

1 pound chicken breasts, lean 1 tablespoon extra virgin olive oil

1 lemon, juiced and zested

cayenne pepper, 1 tblsp

12 teaspoon black pepper, ground

a quarter teaspoon of salt 1/4 cup mustard (Dijon)

1/4 cup chopped rosemary leaves

In a 7 x 11-inch baking dish, place chicken breasts.

In a medium-sized container, combine all ingredients except the chicken.

Pour the marinade over the chicken and turn to coat all sides. For the best flavor, cover and marinate for 1 hour or overnight in the refrigerator.

Preheat oven to 350°F and bake for about 20 minutes.

Before serving, drizzle the remaining sauce over the top.

Information about nutrition: 265 calories, 26.12 grams of protein, 16.27 grams of fat 3.08 g carbohydrate

MEATBALLS WITH HOT CHICKEN

Preparation time: 5 minutes Cooking Time: 21 minutes Serving Size: 14 cup hot sauce is one of the two ingredients.

14 cup grated mozzarella cheese

12 CUP ALMONDFILLER 1 egg 1 pound ground chicken 1 tablespoon mustard To taste, season with salt and black pepper.

Preheat the oven to 4000 degrees Fahrenheit and line a baking tray with parchment paper.

Mix the chicken, black pepper, mustard, flour, mozzarella cheese, salt, and egg in a container. Form meatballs and set them on a baking sheet.

Cook for 16 minutes before adding the hot sauce and baking for another 5 minutes.

Information about nutrition: 487 calories 35 grams of fat net Protein: 31.5g Carbohydrates: 4.3g

CHICKEN ENCHALADAS ON THE KETO DIET

Preparation time: 10 minutes Cooking time: twenty-five minutes Serving Size: 6 ingredients: gluten-free enchilada sauce (6 cups)

Chicken

14 cup fresh cilantro 14 cup chicken broth (chopped) Cups of avocado oil (1 tablespoon) Chicken shreds (cooked) 4 garlic cloves garlic, garlic, garlic, garlic, garlic, garlic (minced)

Assembly

12 tortillas de coco

a quarter cup of green onions (chopped)

Colby jack cheese, 3/4 cup (shredded)

Directions:

In a large pan, heat the oil over medium-high heat. Add the chopped garlic and cook for about one minute, or until fragrant.

Combine rice, 1 cup enchilada sauce (half of the total), chicken, and coriander in a large mixing bowl. Cook for 5 minutes on low heat.

Preheat the oven to 3750 degrees Fahrenheit in the meantime. Using butter, grease a 9x13 baking dish.

Place 14 cup chicken mixture in the center of each tortilla. Roll it up and place it in the baking dish seam side down.

Over the enchiladas, pour the remaining cup of enchilada sauce. Drizzle shredded cheese on top.

Preheat oven to 350°F and bake for ten to twelve minutes. Finish with a sprinkling of green onions.

Information about nutrition: 349 calories, 19 grams of fat 9g Net Carbohydrates 31 g protein

HUMMUS AND LEBANESE CHICKEN KEBABS

Preparation time: 10 minutes + 1 hour marinate

Cooking time: thirty-five minutes

Serving Size: 4\sIngredients:

For the chicken, prepare the following:

1 lemon juice cup 1 tbsp. paprika 1 tbsp. finely chopped thyme 1 tsp. cayenne pepper 1 tsp. cumin powder

4 skinless free-range chicken breasts, cubed 4 skewers for kebabs made of metal

8 garlic cloves, minced Lemon wedges to serve as a garnish

To make the hummus:

1 cup dried chickpeas/1 can chickpeas (soaked overnight) 1 tbsp. Turmeric 1 tsp. Lemon juice tsp. Black pepper Olive oil is a type of oil that comes from

2 tablespoons Paste of tahini

Directions:

In a mixing bowl, combine the lemon juice, garlic, thyme, paprika, cumin, and cayenne pepper.

Using kebab sticks, skewer the chicken cubes (metal).

Brush each side of the chicken with the marinade and refrigerate for as long as possible (the lemon juice will tenderize the meat and means it will be more suitable for the anti-inflammatory diet).

Set the oven to 400°F/200°C/Gas Mark 6 when ready to cook and bake for about 20 minutes, or until the chicken is thoroughly cooked.

To make the hummus, combine all of the ingredients in a blender and process until completely smooth. If the mixture is too thick and lumpy, add a little water to loosen it up.

Serve the chicken kebabs with lemon wedges on the side and hummus on the side.

Information about nutrition: Protein: 61.66 g Fat: 18.55 g Carbohydrates: 42.07 g Calories: 576 kcal Protein: 61.66 g Fat: 18.55 g Carbohydrates: 42.07 g

CHICKEN THIGHS WITH LEMON AND GARLIC

Preparation time: 15 minutes Cooking time: 7–8 hours Serving Size: 4 Ingredients:\steaspoon sea salt

1½ teaspoons garlic powder 2 cups chicken broth\spounds boneless skinless chicken thighs Juice and zest of 1 big lemon

Directions:

Pour the broth into the slow cooker.

In a small container, put the garlic powder, salt, lemon juice, and lemon zest then stir. Baste each chicken thigh with a uniform coating of the mixture. Put the thighs along the bottom of the slow cooker.

Set your cooker on low and secure the lid. Cook for about eight hours, or until the internal temperature of the chicken reaches 165°F on a meat thermometer and the juices run clear,\s before you serve.

Information about nutrition: Calories: 29   Total Fat: 14g
Total Carbohydrates: 3g   Sugar: 0g   Fiber: 0g   \sProtein: 43g
     Sodium: 1,017mg

Chapter Four

LEMON AND HERB CRUSTED CHICKEN FILLETS

Preparation time: 10 minutes Cooking Time: 20 minutes Serving Size: 4

Ingredients:

½ teaspoon garlic powder

½ teaspoon onion

1 cup gluten-free breadcrumbs 1 teaspoon Dijon mustard

1 teaspoon ginger, grated\steaspoon ground black pepper 1 teaspoon lemon peel

1/4 cup lemon juice 2 tablespoons chives\stablespoons fresh thyme, finely chopped 2 tablespoons parsley

2 teaspoons salt

4 Chicken Fillets

Directions:

Preheat your oven to 400 degrees F.

Coat a baking tray with parchment.

Season both sides of chicken fillets. Put skin side down on the\sreadied baking sheet.

Mix the breadcrumbs, chives, thy me, parsley, mustard, ginger, garlic powder, onion powder, and lemon peel in a moderate-sized container.

Drizzle chicken with lemon juice and press the breadcrumb mixture on top of the chicken fillets.

Cook for about twenty minutes.

Information about nutrition: Calories: 1123 kcal   Protein: 196.72 g   Fat: 27.62 g   Carbohydrates: 9.99 g

LEMON-GARLIC CHICKEN AND GREEN BEANS WITH CARAMELIZED ONIONS

Preparation time: 10 minutes Time to Cook: 65 minutes Serving Size: 2\sIngredients:

⅛ tsp. red pepper flakes

¼ cup Golden Ghee, melted\s¼ tsp. paprika

¼ tsp.freshly ground black pepper\stsp. sea salt, plus additional for seasoning 1 yellow onion, quartered\sbig boneless, skinless free-range chicken breasts 2 cups trimmed green beans tbsp. minced garlic

tbsp. extra-virgin olive oil

3 tbsp. freshly squeezed lemon juice

Directions:

In .a medium container or a zipper-top plastic bag, mix the olive oil, lemon juice, garlic, salt, black pepper, paprika, and red pepper flakes.

Place the chicken then coat it in the marinade.

Cover the container or seal the bag then marinate the chicken in your refrigerator for minimum 1 hour, or overnight if possible.

Preheat your oven to 350°F.

Dice 1 of the onion quarters, and chop the remaining 3 quarters into big chunks.

Place the bigger chunks of onion across the bottom of a cast iron or ovenproof frying pan.

Place the green beans, then sprinkle the diced onion above. Put on the top the green beans and onion with the ghee. Place the marinated chicken breasts on the green beans then spoon the rest of the marinade at the chicken. Flavour the dish with a drizzle of sea salt.

Bake the chicken until its internal temperature reaches minimum 165°F, approximately 65 minutes. Serve hot.

Information about nutrition: Calories: 803   Total Fat: 61g   Saturated Fat: 23g   Protein: 53g   Cholesterol: 217mg Carbohydrates: 14g   Fiber: 5g   Net Carbohydrates: 9g

MANGO & LIME BBQ TURKEY

Preparation time: 10 minutes Cooking time: 10 minutes Serving Size: 4\sIngredients:

½ tsp. black pepper

1 medium mango, chopped\s4 boneless, skinless turkey breasts (approximately 1.5-lbs) (approximately 1.5-lbs.) Juice of 2 limes

Zest of 2 limes

Directions:

Mix the lime juice, lime zest, and black pepper in a sealable Ziploc bag. Put in in the turkey, seal bag, and toss to coat.

Set the grill to moderate-high and spray grates with a high heat cooking spray. Grill turkey for five to seven minutes each side or until an internal temperature of approximately 165°F is reached.

While the turkey is grilling, cut up mango.

Remove turkey from grill and place each breast on a serving dish. Top each turkey breast\s

with chopped mango, to decorate. Sprinkle with a little lime juice, if you want. Serve and have fun!

Information about nutrition: Calories: 2110 kcal   Protein: 427.56 g   Fat: 30.95 g   Carbohydrates: 3.94 g

MIDDLE EASTERN SHISH KEBAB

Preparation time: 10 minutes Cooking Time: 20 minutes Serving Size: 5\sIngredients:

½ cup ajran

½ cup tomato sauce 1 tablespoon mustard

2 pounds chicken tenders, cut into bite-sized cubes Turkish spice mix

Directions:

Put chicken tenders with the rest of the ingredients in a ceramic dish. Cover and allow it to marinate for 4 hours in your fridge.

Thread chicken tenders onto skewers and put them on the preheated grill until a golden- brown color is achieved on all sides roughly fifteen minutes.

Serve instantly and enjoy!

Information about nutrition: 274 Calories 10.7g   Fat: 3.3g Carbs: 39.3g   Protein: 0.8g Fiber

MOROCCAN TURKEY TAGINE

Preparation time: 15 minutes Cooking time: 7–8 hours Serving Size: 4 Ingredients:

¼ teaspoon ground coriander

¼ teaspoon ground ginger

¼ teaspoon paprika

½ cup dried apricots

½ cup water

½ red onion, chopped

a quarter teaspoon of salt

1 (14 oz.) can chickpeas, drained

1 (14 oz.) can diced tomatoes 1 tablespoon paste de tomate

1 teaspoon powdered garlic

teaspoon ground turmeric 2 big carrots, finely chopped 2 cups broth of choice

tablespoons raw honey

4 cups boneless, skinless turkey breast chunks Freshly ground black pepper Directions:\sIn your slow cooker, mix the turkey,

tomatoes, chickpeas, carrots, apricots, onion, honey, tomato paste, garlic powder, turmeric, salt, ginger, coriander, paprika, water, and broth, and flavor with pepper. Lightly stir to combine the ingredients.

Set your cooker on low and secure the lid. Cook for about eight hours before you serve.

Information about nutrition: Calories: 428   Total Fat: 5g Total Carbohydrates: 46g   Sugar: 25g   Fiber: 8g   Protein: 49g   Sodium: 983mg

NACHO CHICKEN CASSEROLE

Preparation time: 15 minutes Cooking time: twenty-five minutes Serving Size: 6\sIngredients:\s.25 cup Sour cream

1 cup Green chilies and tomatoes 1 medium Jalapeño pepper\spkg. Frozen cauliflower 1.5tsp. Chili seasoning 1.75lb. Chicken thighs\stbsp. Olive oil\stbsp. Parmesan cheese 4 oz. Cheddar cheese\soz. Cream cheese NEEDED: Immersion blender Pepper and salt (to taste) (to taste)

Directions:

Preheat your oven to 375° Fahrenheit.

Cut the jalapeño into pieces and save for later.

Cutaway the skin and bones from the chicken. Chop it and drizzle using the pepper and salt. Prepare in a frying pan using a portion of olive oil on the med-high temperature setting until browned.

Stir in the sour cream, cream cheese, and ¾ of the cheddar cheese. Stir until melted and blended well. Put in the tomatoes and chilies. Stir then put it all to a baking dish.

Cook the cauliflower in the microwave. Mix in the rest of the cheese with the immersion blender until it looks like mashed potatoes. Season as you wish.

Spread the cauliflower concoction over the casserole and drizzle with the peppers. Bake roughly fifteen to twenty minutes.

Information about nutrition: Calories: 426   Net Carbohydrates: 4.3 g   Total Fat: Content: 32.2 g   Protein: 31 g

SUPREME NUTTY PESTO CHICKEN

Preparation time: 10 minutes Cooking time: 30 minutes Serving Size: 2\s

Ingredients:

12 cup hard cheese (low-fat) (not necessary)

12 cup spinach, uncooked

1 fresh basil bunch in a cup Macadamia nuts, almonds, walnuts, or a mixture 2 tbsp. skinless free-range chicken/turkey breasts olive oil (extra virgin)

Directions:

Preheat the oven to 350 degrees Fahrenheit.

Using a meat pounder, 'thin' each chicken breast into a 1cm thick escalope.

Before adding the other ingredients and a pinch of black pepper to a blender or pestle & mortar, set aside a handful of the nuts and mix until smooth (you can leave this a little lumpy for a rustic feel if you prefer).

If the pesto needs to be loosened, add a little water.

Using the pesto, coat the chicken.

In your oven, bake for at least 30 minutes, or until the chicken is properly done.

Place the remaining nuts on top of each chicken escalope and broil for five minutes to finish with a crispy topping.

Information about nutrition: Protein: 444.61 g Fat: 71.66 g Calories: 2539 kcal 5.99 g carbohydrates

LEGS OF ORANGE CHICKEN

Preparation time: 10 minutes

Cooking Time: 8 Hours Serving Size: 4 components:

14 cup red wine vinegar

12 cup parsley, chopped

1 red onion, peeled and sliced into wedges 4 pieces of chicken leg

5 minced garlic cloves

7 ounces halved canned peaches a sprinkle of black pepper and a pinch of salt 1 orange's juice

1 orange's zest

Combine the orange zest with the orange juice, vinegar, salt, pepper, garlic, onion, peaches, and parsley in a slow cooker. Place the chicken in the pot, mix to combine, cover, and simmer on Low for eight hours. Before serving, divide the mixture into plates.

Enjoy!

Information about nutrition:

251 calories, 4 grams of fat, and 8 grams of fiber 14 grams of carbohydrates 8 g protein CHICKEN STUFFED WITH PANCETTA AND CHEESE

Preparation time: 15 minutes Cooking time: twenty-five minutes Serving Size: 2\sIngredients:

1 minced garlic clove 1 zested lemon, finely chopped shallot tbsp. dried oregano 2 chicken breasts 2 tbsp. extra virgin olive oil

Mascarpone cheese, 4 oz. 4 pancetta slices

Season with salt and black pepper to taste.

In a small frying pan, heat the oil, then sauté the garlic and shallots for approximately three minutes. Combine the salt, black pepper, and lemon zest in a mixing bowl. Transfer to a jar and set aside to cool. Combine the mascarpone cheese and oregano in a mixing bowl.

Cut a pocket in each chicken breast, fill with the cheese mixture, and top with the cut-out chicken. Using a toothpick, secure the ends of each breast with two pancetta pieces.

Place the chicken on a prepared baking sheet and bake for approximately 20 minutes at 380 degrees F.

Information about nutrition: 643 calories 44.5g net fat Carbohydrates: 6.2 g 52.8 g protein

RISOTTO WITH PANCETTA AND CHICKEN

Preparation time: 15 minutes Cooking Time: 15 minutes Serving Size: 2\sIngredients:

12 onion, finely chopped

1 tablespoon zest of lemon 1 tablespoon extra virgin olive oil

1 tablespoon butter (unsalted) 1 teaspoon thyme leaves

white wine, 1/3 cup

12 cup chicken stock; garlic cloves; chopped tablespoon parmesan; grated 2 to 3 slices pancetta; sliced

3/4 cup Arborio rice or risotto

3/4-pound. Diced chicken flesh Season with salt and pepper to taste.

Directions:

Place the oil and butter in the Instant Pot and press the "Sauté" button (*Normal* preset), then wait until the display reads "Hot."

Cook for one to two minutes after adding the onion. In a large mixing bowl, combine the pancetta, chicken, and garlic. Cook for two to three minutes more.

Add the rice and thoroughly combine; the rice must be completely coated in the oil-butter combination. Pour the wine into the pot and scrape the sides. Cook, stirring constantly for two to three minutes. To cancel, use the *Cancel* button.

In a large mixing bowl, combine the chicken stock, thyme, lemon zest, salt, and pepper. Turn the vent to *Sealed* and secure the lid. Set the timer for around six minutes by pressing the *Pressure Cook* (Manual) button and using the *+* or *-*

buttons. Set Pressure to *HIGH* using the *Pressure level* button.

When the timer goes off, push the *Cancel* button and wait for the pressure to naturally dissipate until the float valve lowers.

Open the top and add the parmesan cheese, stirring constantly until it melts. Serve with more parmesan and lemon zest on top.

Information about nutrition: Total Fat: 22.5 g Total Calories: 586 g 23.6 g carbohydrates 45 g protein

SAUSAGE WITH PAN-FRIED CHORIZO

Preparation time: 5 minutes Cooking Time: 15 minutes Serving Size: 4\sIngredients:

12 cup grated Asiago cheese 1 cup pureed tomatoes

1 tablespoon sherry (dry)

1 tbsp extra-virgin extra-virgin olive oil basil (1 teaspoon)

1 teaspoon paste of garlic 1 tsp oregano (oregano)

2 tablespoons fresh coriander, coarsely chopped 4 scallion stalks, chopped 16 ounces smoked turkey chorizo

a pinch of freshly ground black pepper, to taste to taste with sea salt

Oil should be heated in a frying pan over a fairly high heat. Brown the turkey chorizo for about five minutes, crumbling it with a fork.

Except for the cheese, add the other ingredients and simmer for another 10 minutes or until well cooked.

Information about nutrition: Calories: 330 17.2 g fat (4.5 g) Carbohydrates: 34.4 g 1.6 g protein Fiber

SKILLET WITH PAPRIKA CHICKEN AND PANCETTA

Preparation time: 20 minutes Cooking time: 10 minutes Serving Size: 14 tsp sweet paprika (optional) 1 quart chicken broth 1 sliced onion tbsp olive oil

1/3 cup skinless and boneless Dijon mustard chicken breasts 5 pancetta pieces, chopped 2 tablespoons oregano To taste, season with salt and black pepper.

Directions:

Combine the paprika, black pepper, salt, and mustard in a jar. Massage the chicken breasts with this mixture.

Heat a frying pan over medium heat, add the pancetta, and cook until it browns, about 3-4 minutes. Remove to a dish.

Add olive oil to the pancetta grease and cook the chicken breasts for a few minutes on each side. In a large mixing bowl, combine the stock, black pepper, pancetta, salt, and onion. Before serving, sprinkle with oregano.

Calories 323 Calories 323 Calories 323 Calories 323 Calories 323 Calories 3 Net fat: 21g Carbohydrates: 4.8 g 24.5 g protein

CHICKEN WITH PEANUT CRUST

Preparation time: 15 minutes Cooking Time: 15 minutes Serving Size: 2\sIngredients:

12 cup ground peanuts 1 egg boneless and skinless chicken breast halves 3 tablespoons of canola oil

Slices of lemon for decorating To taste, season with salt and black pepper.

Directions:

In one container, whisk the egg; in another, pour the peanuts. Season the chicken, then dip it in the egg and peanuts. Brown the chicken in a skillet over medium heat for a couple of minutes each side.

Place the chicken pieces on a baking sheet, place in the oven, and bake for ten minutes at 360 degrees F. Serve with lemon slices on top.

Calories: 634 g Net Fat: 51 g Net Carbohydrates: 4.7 g 43.6 g protein MOZZARELLA & PESTO CASSEROLE WITH CHICKEN

Preparation time: 10 minutes Cooking Time: 25-30 minutes Serving Size: 8\sIngredients:

a quarter cup of pesto

a quarter-cup to a half-cup of heavy cream

2 pound diced and grilled chicken breasts Cream cheese, 8 oz.

8 oz. mozzarella cubes

8 oz. mozzarella shredded Oil for cooking (as required)

Preheat the oven to 400 degrees Fahrenheit. Using a spritz of cooking oil spray, mist a casserole dish.

Combine the pesto, heavy cream, and softened cream cheese in a large mixing bowl.

In an oiled dish, place the chicken and cubed mozzarella.

Drizzle the shredded mozzarella over the chicken. Preheat the oven to 350°F and bake for about 30 minutes.

Information about nutrition: Net Carbohydrates: 3 g Calories: 451 30 grams of total fat; 38 grams of protein

SALAD WITH PULLED BUFFALO CHICKEN AND BLUE CHEESE

Preparation time: 10 minutes Cooking time: 30 minutes Serving Size: 2\sIngredients:

a quarter cup of buffalo sauce

2 boneless, skinless free-range chicken breasts, split 14 cup chopped red onion, divided 12 cup blue cheese dressing, divided 12 cup crumbled organic blue cheese 4 cups chopped romaine lettuce, split 4 bacon pieces, uncured center-cut

Directions:

Bring a large saucepan of water to a boil over high heat.

Place the chicken breasts in the water, decrease the heat, and simmer for 30 minutes, or until the internal temperature reaches 180°F.

Place the chicken in a container and set aside for ten minutes to cool.

Crisp the bacon strips, on the other hand, in a frying skillet over medium heat for about 3 minutes each side. On a paper towel, drain the bacon. Toss the chicken with the buffalo sauce after shredding it with a fork.

Divide the lettuce into two dishes. Half the pulled chicken, half the blue cheese dressing, blue cheese crumbles, and chopped red onion go on top of each. Before serving, crumble the bacon over the salads.

Calories: 843 Calories: 843 Calories: 843 Calories: 843 Calories: 843 Cal 65g total fat, 14g saturated fat, 59g protein, 156mg cholesterol 6 g carbohydrate, 1 g fiber Carbohydrates (net): 5 g

STUFFED CHICKEN CAPRESE WITH RED PEPPER AND MOZARELLA

Preparation time: 10 minutes Cooking time: 40 minutes Serving Size: 2\sIngredients:

1 mozzarella cheese ball (8 ounces), sliced into 4 pieces 1 cup red peppers, roasted

10 basil leaves, fresh

2 butterflied chicken breasts tbsp extra-virgin olive oil 2 tblsp. seasoning (Italian) black pepper, freshly ground

salt from the sea

Directions:

Preheat the oven to 400 degrees Fahrenheit.

Using parchment paper, line a rimmed baking sheet.

5 basil leaves should be stuffed into each chicken breast.

2 mozzarella slices should be placed within each breast.

The roasted red peppers should be divided into two breasts. Season each breast with salt and pepper and a generous amount of Italian spice. To enclose the filling, close each breast.

Place the breasts on the baking pan and bake for approximately 40 minutes, or until well done. Serve immediately.

Information about nutrition: Total Fat: 30g Calories: 539 5g saturated fat; 63g protein; 152mg cholesterol 4 g carbohydrate, 1 g fiber, 3 g net carbohydrate

CHICKEN THAT HAS BEEN ROASTED

Preparation Time: 60 minutes Cooking Time: 60 minutes Serving Size: 8\sIngredients:

12 tablespoons salt

12 tsp. cayenne pepper

12 teaspoon thyme lbs. whole chicken tbsps. 1 bay leaf garlic cloves Orange peel, coarsely chopped

Prepare the chicken by allowing it to come to room temperature for 1 hour.

Dry the interior and exterior of the chicken with paper towels.

Preheat your oven to 4500 degrees Fahrenheit as soon as you begin making the chicken seasoning.

In a small container, combine the thyme, salt, and pepper.

1/3 of the seasoning should be used to wipe inside the container. Place the garlic, citrus peel, and bay leaf into the chicken.

Tie the legs together and tuck the tips of the wings in. Place the chicken on a roasting pan and season with the remaining spices.

Preheat oven to 1600F and bake for 60 minutes.

Allow fifteen minutes for resting.

Before serving, cut up the roasted chicken.

Enjoy.

Information about nutrition: Protein: 35.48 g Fat: 5.36 g Calories: 201 kcal 0.5 g carbohydrate

WHOLE CHICKEN ROASTED

Preparation time: 20 minutes Cooking time: 1 and 32 minutes Serving Size: 6\sIngredients:

1 grass-fed whole chicken (3 pounds), neck and giblets removed 10 tblsp butter (unsalted)

3 minced garlic cloves

As required, season with salt and black pepper.

Directions:

Preheat the oven to 4000 degrees Fahrenheit. Place an oven rack in the bottom third of the oven.

Using butter, grease a large baking dish.

Cook the butter and garlic in a small saucepan over medium heat for about 1-2 minutes.

Remove the pan from the heat and set it aside to cool for 2 minutes.

Season the interior and outside of the chicken with salt and black pepper in a consistent manner.

Place the chicken breast side up in a prepared baking dish.

Pour the garlic butter all over the chicken, including the insides.

Bake for about 1-112 hours, basting every 20 minutes with the pan juices.

Remove the chicken from the oven and place it on a cutting board for 5-10 minutes before carving.

Before serving, cut into desired size pieces.

Information about nutrition: calorie count: 772 39.1 grams of fat Carbohydrates (net): 0.7g 99 g protein

CHICKEN ROTISSERIE WITH CABBAGE SHREDS

Preparation time: 10 minutes Cooking Time: 0 minutes Serving Size: 2 Ingredients:.5 cup low-carb mayonnaise 1 red onion, 5

1 pound rotisserie chicken, precooked 1 tbsp. extra virgin olive oil

7 ounces cabbage, fresh and green Salt & Pepper

Shred the cabbage and slice the onion into tiny pieces using a sharp kitchen knife.

Place the chicken on a dish with the mayonnaise and a dash of oil. Serve with a salt and pepper dusting.

Calories: 423 g Net Carbohydrates: 6 g Nutritional Information 35 grams of total fat; 17 grams of protein

CHICKEN SALSA VERDE

Preparation time: 15 minutes Cooking time: six to eight hours Serving Size: 4\sIngredients:

1 teaspoon chili powder 1 cup chicken broth 1 tblsp. salt 1 tblsp. green salsa

2 tbsp lime juice, freshly squeezed

4–5 chicken breasts, boneless and skinless (about 2 pounds)

Directions:

Combine the chicken, salsa, broth, lime juice, salt, and chili powder in a slow cooker. To combine the ingredients, stir them together.

Set your cooker on low and secure the lid. Cook for six to eight hours, or until the internal temperature of the chicken reaches 165°F and the juices flow clear when tested with a meat thermometer.

Before serving, shred the chicken with a fork and stir it into the sauce.

Information about nutrition: 318 calories, 8 grams of total fat, 6 grams of total carbohydrate, 2 grams of sugar, 1 gram of fiber, 52 grams of protein 1,510mg sodium

AN EASY TURKEY GOULASH

Preparation time: 15 minutes Preparation time: 45 minutes Serving Size: 4\sIngredients:2 pounds skinless, boneless, and sliced turkey thighs big leek, chopped 2 celery stalks, chopped garlic, minced 2 tablespoons extra virgin olive oil

Directions:

2 olive oil, heated in a clay pot over a moderate to high flame Cook until the leeks are tender and transparent.

Continue to cook the garlic for another half-minute to one minute.

Combine the turkey, celery, and 4 cups of water in a large mixing bowl. Allow the mixture to simmer, partially covered, for around forty minutes after it starts to boil.

Enjoy!

Information about nutrition: Calories: 220 7.4g 2.7g fat 35.5g carbs 1g protein Fiber

Chapter Five

MIX OF SKILLET CHICKEN AND BRUSSELS SPROUTS

Preparation time: 10 minutes Cooking Time: 15 minutes Serving Size: 14 cup chopped walnuts 12 red onion, sliced apple, cored and cut 1 garlic clove, minced 1 tablespoon extra virgin olive oil

12 pound skinless and boneless chicken thighs teaspoons balsamic vinegar 12 ounces shredded brussel sprouts 2 tablespoons thyme, chopped

a sprinkle of black pepper and a pinch of salt

Directions:

Warm the oil in a skillet over medium to high heat, then add the chicken thighs and season with salt, pepper, and thyme.

Cook for 5 minutes on each side before transferring to a container.

Return the pan to a medium heat and add the onion, apple, sprouts, and garlic. Cook for five minutes after tossing the ingredients together. Return the chicken to the pan with the vinegar. Toss in the walnuts, simmer for a few minutes more, then divide into plates before serving.

Enjoy!

Information about nutrition: 211 calories, 4 grams of fat, and 7 grams of fiber 13 Carbohydrates 8 g protein

CHICKEN CACCIATORE IN THE SLOW COOKER

Preparation time: 15 minutes Cooking time: 10 minutes Serving Size: 4

Ingredients:

a quarter teaspoon of red pepper flakes

14 cup extra virgin olive oil

12 oz. red wine

12 CUP TOMATO PUDDING

1 can sodium-free chopped tomatoes (28 oz.) 1 cup mushrooms, sliced

1 tablespoon dried basil 1 onion, diced 1 teaspoon oregano, dry 2 celery stalks, chopped 1 tablespoon garlic, minced

4 boneless chicken breasts, each sliced into three pieces (4 ounces)

Directions:

Cook the chicken in a skillet. Warm the olive oil in a frying pan over medium to high heat. Place the chicken breasts in the pan and brown them for about ten minutes, flipping once.

In a slow cooker, prepare the dish. Combine the chicken, onion, celery, mushrooms, garlic, tomatoes, red wine, tomato paste, basil, oregano, and red pepper flakes in a slow cooker. Cook for three to four hours on high or six to eight hours on low, until the chicken is thoroughly cooked and tender.

Serve. Serve immediately by dividing the chicken and sauce across four bowls.

Information about nutrition: 383 calories 26g total fat 11g total carbohydrates; 4g fiber 7g net carbohydrates; 116mg sodium; 26g protein

CHICKEN FAJITAS IN THE SLOW COOKER

Preparation time: 15 minutes Cooking time: 7–8 hours Serving Size: 4 components:

1 can chopped tomatoes (14.5 oz.)

1 can (4 oz.) Green chiles, Hatch 1 large onion, peeled and chopped 1 green bell pepper, seeded and peeled 1 seeded and sliced red bell pepper

paprika, 1 teaspoon 1 teaspoon salt, seeded and sliced yellow bell pepper 112 tblsp garlic powder pound boneless, skinless chicken breast 112 tablespoons cumin chili powder (about 2 tablespoons) black pepper, freshly ground 1 lime's juice

a pinch of cayenne

Directions:

Combine the diced tomatoes, chiles, garlic powder, chili powder, cumin, paprika, salt, lime juice, and cayenne in a medium-sized container, season with black pepper, and stir. Pour half of the diced tomato mixture into the slow cooker's bottom.

Half of the red, green, and yellow bell peppers, as well as half of the onion, should be layered over the tomatoes in the slow cooker.

On top of the peppers and onions, place the chicken.

Add the remaining red, green, and yellow bell peppers and onions to the chicken. Pour the remaining tomato sauce on top.

Set your cooker on low and secure the lid. Before serving, cook the chicken for approximately eight hours, or until the internal temperature reaches 165°F on a meat thermometer and the juices flow clear.

Information about nutrition: 310 calories, 5 grams of total fat, 19 grams of total carbohydrate, 7 grams of sugar, 4 grams of fiber, 46 grams of protein 1,541mg sodium

JERK CHICKEN IN A SLOW COOKER

Preparation time: 10 minutes

Cooking Time: 5 Hours Serving Size: 4 components:

1 teaspoon black pepper (2 g) teaspoon (2 g) teaspoons cayenne pepper (3 g) thyme, dried

4 g white pepper (2 teaspoons)

2 tablespoons onion powder (5 g)

6 g garlic powder (2 tablespoons)

4 tablespoons salt (20 g)

8 chicken wings and 4 tablespoons (9 g) paprika chicken drumsticks

Directions:

To prepare a rub for the chicken, combine all of the spices in a jar and stir well.

Rinse the chicken flesh in cold water for a few minutes. Place the rinsed chicken flesh in the rub container and thoroughly massage the spices into the meat, particularly beneath the skin.

Place each piece of chicken in the slow cooker, spiced on both sides (no liquid required).

Cook for about five hours on low or until the chicken flesh slips off the bone in the slow cooker.

Information about nutrition: 480 calories, 30 grams of fat Carbohydrates (net): 4 g 45 g protein

GARLIC LIME TARTAR SAUCE WITH SPICY ALMOND CHICKEN STRIPS

Preparation time: 10 minutes Cooking time: 10 minutes Serving Size: 4 components:

Sticks of chicken:

12 CUP ALMON FLOUR, BLANCHED

12 CUP COCONUT OLIVE OIL

12 teaspoon cayenne pepper, ground

12 pound chicken breast, cut into 1x5-inch chunks 1 teaspoon kosher salt

1/4 cup basil leaves, dried

1/4 teaspoon black pepper, freshly ground 2 free-range organic eggs, whisked

Garlic Lime Tartar Sauce: 3 garlic cloves, coarsely chopped

a quarter teaspoon of salt

12 tablespoon relish (dill pickle) 1 tablespoon mayonnaise

1 tablespoon onion flakes (dry) 1 teaspoon powdered garlic

lime juice, 1 tbsp

Directions:

To make the tartar sauce, whisk together all of the ingredients until smooth. Refrigerate for at least 30 minutes before serving.

In a medium-sized container, whisk together the eggs. Combine almond flour, cayenne pepper, basil, garlic, salt, and pepper in a separate container.

Dip chicken strips in the egg, then in the flour mixture; coat well and arrange on a platter.

In a deep frying pan over medium to high heat, melt some coconut oil. Cook for at least two minutes on each side, until well-browned, using half of the chicken strips. Make sure there's enough space around the chicken strips so they don't become too crowded.

Using paper towels on a plate, drain the sticks. Cook the remaining half of the chicken strips in another 1/4 cup coconut oil. Serve with the Garlic Lime Tartar Sauce that has been made.

Information about nutrition: Protein: 94.15 g Fat: 75.01 g Calories: 1092 kcal 7.5 g carbohydrate

CHICKEN TANGY BARBECUE

Preparation time: 15 minutes Cooking time: 3-4 hours Serving Size: 4 components:

2 quarts Tangy Apple Cider Vinegar Barbecue Sauce

4- 5 boneless, skinless chicken breasts (2 lb.)

Directions:

Combine the chicken and barbecue sauce in a slow cooker. Stir until the sauce is evenly distributed among the chicken breasts.

Set your stove on high and secure the lid. Cook for three to four hours, or until the juices flow clear and the internal temperature of the chicken reaches 165°F on a meat thermometer.

Before serving, shred the chicken with a fork and stir it into the sauce.

Information about nutrition: calorie count: 412 13 g total fat Sugar: 19g Total Carbohydrates: 22g Protein: 51g Fiber: 0g Fiber: 0g Fiber: 0g Fiber: 0g Fiber: 0g Fiber: 0 766mg sodium

SCALLIONS AND TANGY CHICKEN

Preparation time: 10 minutes Cooking time: 40 minutes 4 servings (about)

Ingredients:

1 pound chicken drumettes 1 garlic clove, sliced

1 tablespoon chopped fresh scallions white wine, 2 teaspoons

3 teaspoons melted butter

Directions:

Place the chicken drumettes in a baking tray lined with foil. Brush the surface with melted butter.

Combine the garlic and wine in a mixing bowl. To taste, season with salt and black pepper. Preheat the oven to 400 degrees F and bake for about 30 minutes, or until the internal temperature reaches 165 degrees F.

Serve with scallions on top and enjoy!

Calories in this recipe: 209 12.2g 0.4g fat 23.2g carbs 1.9g protein Fiber

ROASTED BALSAMIC TURNIPS WITH TARRAGON CHICKEN

Preparation time: 10 minutes Cooking Time: 50 minutes Serving Size: 2-4 pound chicken thighs Ingredients: 1 tablespoon balsamic vinaigrette 1 tablespoon tarragon 1 pound turnips, wedged 2 tbsp. extra virgin olive oil

To taste, season with salt and black pepper.

Preheat the oven to 400 degrees Fahrenheit and grease a baking dish with olive oil. Turnips should be cooked for approximately ten minutes in boiling water, then drained and saved for later. In a baking dish, combine the chicken and turnips.

Drizzle tarragon, black pepper, and salt over the top. For a little more than half an hour, roast. Remove the baking dish, drizzle the balsamic vinegar over the turnip wedges, and return to the oven for another five minutes.

Information about nutrition: 383 calories, 26 grams of fat Net Protein: 21.3g Carbohydrates: 9.5g

WRAPS OF THE TURKEY CLUB

Preparation time: 5 minutes Cooking time: 5 minutes Serving Size: 12 slice sharp American cheese, first ingredient (cut deli-thin) 1 whole wheat tortilla or flatbread wrap

ranch yogurt dressing (tbsp.) 2 fried bacon slices tomato slices smoked turkey (2 oz) (cut deli-thin) lettuce romaine (or baby spinach)

To begin, apply ranch dressing evenly over the middle of the wrap or tortilla.

Layer the turkey, cheese, bacon, tomato, and lettuce on top of that (or spinach).

To finish, fold each edge of the wrap or tortilla in half and roll it up.

Information about nutrition: TURKEY CRUST MEATZA CALORIES: 791 kcal PROTEIN: 31.84 g FAT: 63.37 g CARBS: 22.53 g

Preparation time: 15 minutes Cooking time: thirty-five minutes Serving Size: 4\sIngredients:

12 pound turkey ground

1 cup grated Mozzarella cheese 1 teaspoon pizza seasoning

tomato slices, chopped Bacon from Canada

Combine the ground turkey and cheese in a mixing bowl; season with salt and black pepper and toss until thoroughly combined.

Fill a foil-lined baking sheet halfway with the mixture. Preheat the oven to 380 degrees F and bake for approximately 25 minutes.

Canadian bacon, tomato, and pizza spice mix go on top of the dough. Continue to bake for another 8 minutes.

Allow for a few minutes to rest before cutting and serving. Enjoy!

360 calories, 22.7 grams of fat, 5.9 grams of carbs, 32.6 grams of sugar 0.7 g protein Fiber

PATE WITH TURKEY HAM AND MOZZARELLA

Preparation time: 10 minutes Cooking Time: 0 minutes Serving Size: 6\sIngredients:

flaxseed meal, 2 tblsp.

2 teaspoons finely chopped fresh parsley sunflower seeds, 2 teaspoons

4 oz. crumbled mozzarella cheese 4 oz. chopped turkey ham

In a food processor, thoroughly combine all of the ingredients, except the sunflower seeds.

Fill a serving pitcher halfway with the mixture and top with the sunflower seeds.

212 calories, 18.8 grams of fat, 10.6 grams of carbohydrates, and 1.6 grams of protein Fiber

MEATBALLS WITH TURKEY AND SPAGHETTI SQUASH

Preparation time: 15 minutes Cooking time: 7–8 hours Serving Size: 4\sIngredients:

12 tbsp. minced white onion

12 teaspoon basil leaves, dried

12 teaspoon oregano, dry

a quarter teaspoon of garlic powder

a quarter teaspoon of salt

1 (fifteen-ounce) can tomatoes, diced 1 large whisked egg

1 pound turkey ground

1 spaghetti squash, seeds and split along the length 1 teaspoon powdered garlic

To make the meatballs, combine the following ingredients in a large mixing bowl.

To make the sauce:

black pepper, freshly ground

Directions:

1. Place the squash halves cut-side down on the bottom of your slow cooker.

To prepare the sauce, follow these steps:

On the bottom of the slow cooker, pour the chopped tomatoes around the squash.

Add the garlic powder, oregano, and salt to taste.

To create the meatballs, follow these steps:

Combine the turkey, egg, onion, garlic powder, salt, oregano, and basil in a medium-sized container and season with pepper. Form the turkey mixture into 12 balls and place them around the spaghetti squash in the slow cooker.

Set your cooker on low and secure the lid. Cook for 6 to 7 hours at a low temperature.

Transfer the squash to a cutting board and shred it with a fork into spaghetti-like strands. Before serving, combine the strands with the tomato sauce and top with the meatballs.

Information about nutrition: calorie count: 253 8 g total fat 22 g total carbohydrate, 4 g sugar 1 g fiber, 24 g protein 948 mg sodium

SLOPPY JOES WITH TURKEY

Preparation time: 15 minutes Cooking time: four to six hours Serving Size: 4\sIngredients:

12 medium sliced sweet onion

12 finely sliced red bell pepper

12 teaspoon oregano, dry

a quarter teaspoon of garlic powder

a quarter teaspoon of salt 1 carrot, finely minced

1 minced celery stalk 1 pound turkey ground

1 tbsp extra-virgin extra-virgin olive oil 1 teaspoon of maple syrup

a tablespoon of chili powder 1 tablespoon apple cider vinegar 1 teaspoon Dijon mustard Tomato paste (six tablespoons)

Directions:

Combine the turkey, celery, carrot, onion, red bell pepper, tomato paste, vinegar, maple syrup, mustard, chili powder, garlic powder, salt, and oregano in a slow cooker. As the turkey merges with the other ingredients, break it up into smaller bits with a large spoon.

Set your cooker on low and secure the lid. Cook for four to six hours, stirring often before serving.

Information about nutrition: calorie count: 251 12 g total fat Sugar: 9g Total Carbohydrates: 14g 3 g of fiber 24 g protein 690 mg sodium

GINGER SAUCE ON TURMERIC CHICKEN WINGS

Preparation time: 5 minutes Cooking Time: 20 minutes Serving Size: 2-4

Ingredients:

a third of a cup of chopped cilantro 1 tablespoon thyme leaves

1 pepper, jalapeo

1 pound cut-in-half chicken wings 1 tablespoon cumin

turmeric, 1 tbsp.

tbsp. olive oil tbsp. water

1 tablespoon grated fresh ginger 12 lime juice

To taste, season with salt and black pepper.

Directions:

Combine 1 tablespoon ginger, cumin, salt, half of the olive oil, black pepper, turmeric, and cilantro in a jar. Place the chicken wings pieces in the bowl, toss to coat, and chill for approximately 20 minutes.

Raise the temperature of the grill to high. Remove the wings from the marinade, drain, and grill for approximately 20 minutes, flipping once or twice, before setting them aside.

Blend together the thyme, remaining ginger, salt, jalapeño pepper, black pepper, lime juice, the remaining olive oil, and water in a blender until smooth. Serve the chicken wings with the sauce on top.

Information about nutrition: 253 calories 16.1 g net fat 4.1 g carbs 21.7 g protein

CHICKEN WITH TURNIP GREENS AND ARTICHOKE

Preparation time: 5 minutes Cooking time: 30 minutes Serving Size: 2\sIngredients:

14 cup grated Pecorino cheese

12 tablespoons garlic powder

12 tablespoons onion powder turnip greens, 1 cup

2 breasts of chicken

2 oz. shredded Monterrey Jack cheese cream cheese, 4 oz.

4 oz. chopped canned artichoke hearts To taste, season with salt and black pepper.

Directions:

Place the chicken breasts in a baking dish lined with parchment paper. Flavor it with black pepper and salt. Set in your oven at 350 F and bake for a little more than half an hour.

In a container, mix the artichokes with onion powder, Pecorino cheese, salt, turnip greens, cream cheese, garlic powder, and black pepper.

Take off the chicken from the oven, cut each piece in half, split artichokes mixture on top, spread with Monterrey cheese, and bake for 5 more minutes.

Information about nutrition: Calories 443   Fat: 24.5g Net Carbs: 4.2g   Protein: 35.4g

TUSCAN CHICKEN SAUTE

Preparation time: 10 minutes Cooking time: thirty-five minutes Serving Size: 4\sIngredients:

¼ cup cut Kalamata olives

½ cup heavy (whipping) cream

½ cup shredded Asiago cheese

½ teaspoon dried basil

¾ cup chicken stock 1 cup fresh spinach

1 pound boneless chicken breasts, each cut into three pieces

1 tablespoon garlic, minced

1 teaspoon dried oregano 3 tablespoons olive oil

Freshly ground black pepper, for seasoning Sea salt, for seasoning

Directions:

Prepare the chicken. Pat, the chicken, breasts dry and lightly flavor them with salt and pepper.

Sauté the chicken. In a big frying pan on moderate to high heat, warm the olive oil. Put in the chicken and sauté until it is golden brown and just thoroughly cooked, approximately fifteen minutes in total. Move the chicken to a plate and set it aside.

Make the sauce. Place the garlic to the frying pan, then sauté until it's softened about two minutes. Mix in the chicken stock, oregano, and basil, scraping up any browned bits in the frying pan. Bring to its boiling point, then decrease the heat to low and simmer until the sauce is reduced by about one-quarter, approximately ten minutes.

Finish the dish. Mix in the cream, Asiago, and simmer while stirring the sauce regularly, until it has become thick about five minutes. Put back the chicken to the frying pan together with any collected juices. Mix in the spinach and olives and simmer until the spinach is wilted about two minutes.

Serve. Split the chicken and sauce between four plates and serve it instantly.

Nutritional Info: Calories: 483 Total fat: 38g Total carbs: 5g Fiber: 1g; Net carbs: 3g

Sodium: 332mg   Protein: 31g

VODKA DUCK FILLETS

Time To Prepare: five minutes Time to Cook: 15 minutes Yield: Servings 4

Ingredients:

½ cup sour cream

½ teaspoon ground bay leaf 1 ½ cups turkey stock

tablespoon lard, room temperature 1 teaspoon mixed peppercorns

ounces vodka

tablespoons Worcestershire sauce 4 duck fillets

green onions, chopped

Salt and cayenne pepper, to taste

Directions:

Melt the lard in a frying pan that is preheated on moderate to high heat. Sear the duck fillets, flipping over once, for four to six minutes.

Now, put in the rest of the ingredients, apart from for the sour cream, to the frying pan. Cook, partly covered, for another seven minutes.

Serve warm, decorated with sour cream. Enjoy!

Nutritional Info: 351 Calories 24.7g   Fat: 6.6g   Carbs: 22.1g Protein

Chapter Six

CHILI BLANCA WITH WHITE BEANS AND CHICKEN

fifteen minutes to prepare Cooking Time: 30 min Servings Count 4-5\sIngredients:

12 cup fresh or frozen corn kernels

12 pound boneless skinless chicken tenders or boneless chicken breasts 12 cup of water

1 can (15 oz.) white or Great Northern beans, rinsed and drained 1 garlic clove, peeled and minced

1 cup grated Monterey Jack cheese 1 sliced small onion

1 tbsp olive oil extra-virgin

1 tablespoon chopped fresh cilantro 1 teaspoon cayenne pepper

a teaspoon of cumin powder ounces of green chiles, canned cayenne pepper, a sprinkle season with pepper to taste

To taste, season with salt

Directions:

Season the chicken with salt and pepper.

Using high heat, place a frying pan on the stove. Pour in the oil. When the oil is hot, add the chicken and cook until it is brown.

Reduce the heat to a medium setting. Sauté the garlic and onion until they are soft.

Combine the corn, beans, green chilies, water, cumin powder, chili powder, salt, and cayenne pepper in a large mixing bowl. Cook for around 20 minutes on low heat.

Pour into serving dishes. Before serving, garnish with cheese and cilantro.

Information about the calories: 243 calories per serving; 20.57 grams of protein; 13.94 grams of fat 11.96 g carbohydrate

CHILI WITH WHITE BEANS, CHICKEN, AND APPLE CIDER

15 minutes to prepare 7–8 hours to cook Servings Count 4\sIngredients:

a quarter-cup of apple cider vinegar

14 teaspoon cinnamon powder

12 teaspoon cumin powder

1 can chopped tomatoes (15 oz.)

1 apple cider cup

1 medium sliced onion

1 tbsp olive oil extra-virgin 1 teaspoon cayenne pepper

(fifteen-ounce cans) white navy beans, cleaned and drained teaspoon sea salt 2 bay leaves 2 tblsp garlic powder 2 cups Bone broth from chickens or store-bought chicken broth

3 cups cooked chicken, chopped (see "Rotisserie" Chicken Basics) Black pepper, freshly ground

1 tblsp. cayenne

Directions:

Combine the chicken, beans, onion, tomatoes, broth, cider, bay leaves, olive oil, garlic powder, chili powder, salt, cumin, cinnamon, and cayenne pepper in a slow cooker. Season with black pepper.

Set your cooker's lid to low and lock it in place. Allow for an eight-hour cooking time.

Remove the bay leaves and toss them out. Before serving, stir in the apple cider vinegar until well combined.

Information about the calories: calorie count: 469 8 grams total fat 46 g total carbohydrate, 13 g sugar, 9 g fiber, 51 g protein Sodium: 1,047 milligrams

CHICKEN WITH VEGETABLES IN THE WINTER

Preparation time: 5 min Cooking Time: 30 min Servings Count 2\sIngredients:

1 leaf of bay

1 grated carrot

1 pound chicken breasts, chopped 1 turnip, chopped cups chicken stock 1 cup green beans, diced 1 onion, chopped 1 parsnip, chopped

2 quarts whipped cream olive oil, 2 tbsp.

2 tsp chopped fresh thyme To taste, season with salt and pepper.

Directions:

Warm the olive oil in a pan over medium heat. After three minutes of sautéing the onion, add the stock, carrot, turnip, parsnip, chicken, and bay leaf. Bring to a boil, then reduce to a low heat for approximately 20 minutes.

Cook for seven minutes after adding the asparagus. To serve, discard the bay leaf, stir in the whipped cream, adjust the salt, and top with fresh thyme. Information about the calories: 483 calories 32.5g fat (net) Carbohydrates: 6.9 g 33 g protein

BEET HUMMUS HUMMUS HUMMUS HUMMUS

Preparation time: 5 min 0 minutes to prepare Servings Count 2\sIngredients:

14 teaspoon chili powder

12 cup extra virgin olive oil

12 teaspoon oregano

12 teaspoon salt

12 teaspoon cumin

a third of a cup of chickpeas a single garlic clove

1 fresh ginger nub 1 roasted beet (skinless) 1 tsp curry powder

1 tbsp maple syrup

sunflower seeds (tbsp.) One lemon's juice

Instructions: In a food processor, combine all of the ingredients until smooth, then garnish with sunflower seeds.

Enjoy!

Information about the calories: 423 calories per serving; 13.98 grams of protein; 24.26 grams of fat 40.13 g carbohydrates

STIR FRY BROCCOLI AND BLACK BEANS

fifteen minutes to prepare Cooking time: fifteen minutes Servings Count 4 ingredients: 1 tablespoon sesame oil garlic cloves, finely chopped 2 cups black beans, cooked

2 tablespoons finely chopped ginger Broccoli florets, 4 cups

sesame seeds, 4 tblsp. a generous teaspoon of red chili flakes turmeric powder, a pinch

to flavor lime juice (not necessary) To taste, season with salt Pour enough water into the large frying pan to cover the bottom by an inch. On the deep frying pan, place a strainer. Broccoli florets should be placed in the strainer. Broccoli should be steamed for around six minutes.

Preheat a large frying pan over medium heat. Pour sesame oil into the pan. Add sesame seeds, chili flakes, ginger, garlic, turmeric powder, and salt to the hot oil. Sauté for 2 minutes, or until fragrant.

Sauté the steamed broccoli and black beans until they are well cooked.

Stir in the lime juice.

Warm it up and serve.

Information about the calories: 196 calories per serving; 11.2 grams of protein; 7.25 grams of fat 23.45 g carbohydrate

ONIONS AND CARAMELIZED PEARS

Preparation time: 5 min Cooking Time: 35 min Servings Count 4 Ingredients: 1 tablespoon extra virgin olive oil

hard red pears, quartered and cored 2 red onions, peeled and sliced into wedges

Season with salt and pepper to taste.

Preheat the oven to 425 degrees Fahrenheit.

Sprinkle olive oil over the pears and onion on a baking dish.

Season to taste with salt and pepper.

Bake for a little more than half an hour in your oven.

Enjoy your meal!

Calories: 101; Fat: 4g; Carbohydrates: 0; Protein: 0; Carbohydrates: 0; Carbohydrates: 0; 17 g Carbohydrates 1 gram of protein

MASH OF CAULIFLOWER AND BROCCOLI

Preparation time: 5 min Cooking Time: 10 min Servings Count 6 Ingredients: 1 large cauliflower head, sliced into bits 1 floret of broccoli from a small head 1 tsp sodium

3 tbsp olive oil (extra virgin) salt and pepper to taste

Directions:

Put some oil in a saucepan and heat it up.

Place the cauliflower and broccoli in the pot.

To taste, season with salt and pepper.

Continue stirring until the vegetables are tender.

If necessary, add water.

Use a food processor or a potato masher to purée the veggies after they've been cooked.

Enjoy your meal!

Information about the calories: calorie count: 39 3 g of fat 2 g Carbohydrates 0.89 g protein

PLATTER WITH CILANTRO AND AVOCADO

fifteen minutes to prepare 0 minutes to prepare Servings Count 6 ingredients: 14 cup chopped fresh cilantro 12 lime juice

1 large ripe tomato, chopped green bell pepper, chopped 1 sweet onion, peeled, pitted, and diced avocados Season with salt and pepper as needed.

Place the onion, bell pepper, tomato, avocados, lime, and cilantro in a medium-sized container.

Toss everything together well.

Depending on your preference, season with salt and pepper.

Enjoy your meal!

Information about the calories: Calories: 126 Fat grams: 10 10 g Carbohydrates 2 g protien

COUSCOUS CITRUS WITH HERBS

Preparation time: 5 min Cooking time: fifteen minutes Servings Count 2\sIngredients:

12 teaspoon butter 14 cup water 14 orange, diced

1 teaspoon spices (Italian) a third of a cup of couscous

a third teaspoon of salt

a quarter-cup of orange juice

Fill the pan halfway with water and orange juice.

Combine the orange, Italian seasoning, and salt in a mixing bowl.

Bring the liquid to a boil, then remove from the heat.

Add the butter and couscous to the pan. Close the cover after fully stirring.

Allow 10 minutes for the couscous to rest.

Information about the calories: 149 calories Carbs: 28.5 Carbs: 1.9 Fat: 1.9 Fiber: 2.1 Fat: 1.9 Fat: 1.9 Fat: 1.9 Fat: 1.9 Fat: 1.9 Fat: 1.9 Fat: 4.1 g protein

BEANS WITH SPINACH AND GARBANZO

Preparation time: 5–10 minutes

Cooking time: 0 minutes Servings Count 4 items:

12 onion (diced)

1 tablespoon olive oil 12 teaspoon cumin

12 ounces garbanzo beans 10 ounces spinach, diced

Fill a frying pan halfway with olive oil and set aside.

Set the temperature to medium to low.

Cook for five minutes after adding the onions and garbanzo beans.

Cumin, garbanzo beans, spinach, and sunflower seeds are added to the mix.

Gently crush with a spoon.

Cook with care.

Enjoy your meal!

Information about the calories: calorie count: 90 4 g of fat 11 g carbohydrate, 4 g protein

SALAD WITH COUSCOUS

fifteen minutes to prepare Cooking time: six minutes Servings Count 4\sIngredients:

14 teaspoon black pepper, ground

34 teaspoon coriander powder

12 tsp sodium

a quarter teaspoon of paprika

a quarter teaspoon of turmeric 1 tablespoon unsalted butter

2 oz. canned chickpeas, drained 1 cup chopped fresh arugula

2 oz. chopped sun-dried tomatoes 1 oz. crumbled Feta cheese

1 tblsp. rapeseed oil a third of a cup of couscous

1/3 cup stock made from chicken

Prepare the chicken stock by bringing it to a boil.

Combine the couscous, black pepper, ground coriander, salt, paprika, and turmeric in a mixing bowl. Add the chickpeas and the butter. Close the cover after thoroughly mixing the ingredients.

Allow six minutes for the couscous to soak in the heated chicken broth.

Meanwhile, combine arugula, sun-dried tomatoes, and Feta cheese in a mixing container.

Combine the cooked couscous and canola oil in a mixing bowl.

Toss the salad well.

Information about the calories: calorie count: 18 calorie count: 18 calorie count: 18 calorie count: 9 % fat Carbs: 21.1 Fiber:

3.6 Fiber: 3.6 Fiber: 3.6 Fiber: 3.6 Fiber: 3.6 Fiber: 3.6 Fiber: 3.6 Fiber 6 g protein

POLENTA CREAMY

Preparation time: 8 minutes Cooking Time: 45 min Servings Count 4\sIngredients:

12 cup heavy cream 12 cup of water 1 polenta cup

1/3 cup grated Parmesan 2 cups stock (chicken)

Place the polenta in a saucepan and bring to a boil.

In a large mixing bowl, combine the water, chicken stock, cream, and Parmesan cheese. Mix the polenta well.

Preheat the oven to 355 degrees Fahrenheit.

Preheat the oven to 350°F and bake the polenta for 45 minutes.

Before serving, carefully stir together the prepared food with the spoon.

Calories: 208; Fat: 5.3; Fiber: 1; Carbs: 32.2; Protein: 8; Calories: 208; Fat: 5.3; Fiber: 1; Carbs: 32.2; Protein: 8 CRISPY CORN

Preparation time: 8 minutes Cooking Time: 5 min Servings Count 3\sIngredients:

12 teaspoon paprika powder

12 tblsp salt 34 tblsp chili powder 1 cup kernels of corn

1 tablespoon flour (coconut) 1 teaspoon of water

a third of a cup of canola oil

Instructions: Combine corn kernels, salt, and coconut flour in a mixing container.

Pour in the water and stir in the corn with a spoon.

Heat up the canola oil in the frying pan.

Place the corn kernels mixture in the oven and cook for four minutes. It should be stirred every now and again.

When the corn kernels are crispy, transfer them to the dish and dry them with a paper towel.

Add the chili pepper and paprika powder. Mix everything up well.

Information about the calories: 179 calories, fifteen grams of fat Carbs: 11.3 g Fiber: 2.4 g Fiber: 2.4 g Fiber: 2.4 g Fiber: 2.4 g Fiber: 2.1 CUCUMBER YOGURT SALAD WITH MINT PROTEIN

fifteen minutes to prepare 0 minutes to prepare Servings Count 2\sIngredients:

14 cup coconut milk (organic)

14 cup mint leaves (organic)

14 teaspoon Himalayan pink salt

12 cup organic red onion, chopped 1 tbsp extra virgin olive oil 1 tbsp organic plain goat yogurt 1 tablespoon fresh organic lime juice 1 teaspoon organic dill weed sliced organic cucumbers

Cut the red onion, dill, cucumbers, and mint into small pieces and combine them in a large container.

Blend until they're completely smooth.

Toss the cucumber salad with the dressing and combine well. Serve after chilling for at least 1 hour.

Enjoy!

Calories: 207 kcal Protein: 6.9 g Fat: 13.87 g Carbohydrates: 18.04 g Nutritional Information: Calories: 207 kcal Protein: 6.9 g Fat: 13.87 g Carbohydrates: 18.04 g

RICE WITH WHEATBERRY CURRY

fifteen minutes to prepare

Cooking time: 1 hour 15 minutes

Servings Count 5\sIngredients:

14 cup of milk

rice (12 cup)

wheat berries (1 cup)

1 teaspoon curry powder 1 tsp sodium

4 tablespoons extra virgin olive oil 6 cups stock (chicken) In a skillet, combine the wheatberries and chicken stock.

Cook the mixture for an hour over medium heat with the lid closed.

After that, add the rice, olive oil, and salt.

Completely combine all ingredients.

Combine the milk and curry paste in a mixing bowl.

In the rice-wheatberry combination, pour in the curry liquid and stir well.

Cook the food for 15 minutes with the lid closed.

When the rice is done, the rest of the dinner is ready.

Information about the calories: 232 cals 15 pounds of fat Carbohydrates: 23.5 Fiber: 1.4 Protein: 3.9

SALAD WITH FARRO AND ARUGULA

fifteen minutes to prepare Cooking Time: 35 min Servings Count 2\sIngredients:

12 c. farro

12 tsp black pepper, freshly ground

12 teaspoon seasoning (Italian)

12 teaspoon extra virgin olive oil

12 cup stock (chicken) 1 tbsp lemon juice 1 cucumber, diced 1 teaspoon salt 1 cup chopped arugula

Directions: Combine farro, salt, and chicken stock in a skillet and stir to combine.

Boil for a little more than half an hour with the lid closed.

Meanwhile, combine the other ingredients in the salad container.

Bring the farro to room temperature before adding it to the salad container.

Toss the salad well.

Calories 92 Calories 92 Calories 92 Calories 92 Calories 92 Calories 2.3 g of fat, 2 g of fiber Carbohydrates: 15.6 FETA: 3.9 protein SALAD WITH CHEESE

fifteen minutes to prepare 0 minutes to prepare Servings Count 2 Ingredients: 1 tablespoon olive oil (extra virgin) cucumbers, 1 teaspoon balsamic vinegar

feta cheese, 30 g 4 green onions

4 tomatillos

Salt

Cucumbers and tomatoes should be chopped into cubes.

Onions should be sliced thinly.

Feta cheese should be crushed.

Tomatoes, onions, and cucumbers should all be mixed together.

Combine the olive oil, vinegar, and a pinch of salt in a small mixing bowl.

feta cheese should be added.

Have fun eating!

Calories: 221 kcal Protein: 9.24 g Fat: 13.84 g Carbohydrates: 17.18 g Nutritional Information: Calories: 221 kcal Protein: 9.24 g Fat: 13.84 g

STRAWBERRY SALSA WITH FRESH STRAWBERRY

fifteen minutes to prepare 0 minutes to prepare Yield: 6–8 people

Ingredients:

14 c. lime juice, freshly squeezed

12 cup cilantro, chopped

12 cup coarsely chopped red onion 12 teaspoon grated lime zest 1-2 deseeded jalapeos 2 pounds fresh ripe strawberries, hulled and diced 2 kiwis, peeled and chopped 2 tsp. honey (raw)

In a large mixing bowl, whisk together lime juice, lime zest, and honey.

Add the rest of the ingredients and stir well. Cover and leave aside for a few minutes to allow the flavors to meld.

Calories: 119 kcal Protein: 9.26 g Fat: 4.38 g Carbohydrates: 11.73 g Nutritional Information: Calories: 119 kcal Protein: 9.26 g Fat: 4.38 gCHILI BLANCA WITH WHITE BEANS AND CHICKEN

fifteen minutes to prepare Cooking Time: 30 min Servings Count 4-5\sIngredients:

12 cup fresh or frozen corn kernels

12 pound boneless skinless chicken tenders or boneless chicken breasts 12 cup of water

1 can (15 oz.) white or Great Northern beans, rinsed and drained 1 garlic clove, peeled and minced

1 cup grated Monterey Jack cheese 1 sliced small onion

1 tbsp olive oil extra-virgin

1 tablespoon chopped fresh cilantro 1 teaspoon cayenne pepper

a teaspoon of cumin powder ounces of green chiles, canned cayenne pepper, a sprinkle season with pepper to taste

To taste, season with salt

Directions:

Season the chicken with salt and pepper.

Using high heat, place a frying pan on the stove. Pour in the oil. When the oil is hot, add the chicken and cook until it is brown.

Reduce the heat to a medium setting. Sauté the garlic and onion until they are soft.

Combine the corn, beans, green chilies, water, cumin powder, chili powder, salt, and cayenne pepper in a large mixing bowl. Cook for around 20 minutes on low heat.

Pour into serving dishes. Before serving, garnish with cheese and cilantro.

Information about the calories: 243 calories per serving; 20.57 grams of protein; 13.94 grams of fat 11.96 g carbohydrate

CHILI WITH WHITE BEANS, CHICKEN, AND APPLE CIDER

15 minutes to prepare 7–8 hours to cook Servings Count 4\sIngredients:

a quarter-cup of apple cider vinegar

14 teaspoon cinnamon powder

12 teaspoon cumin powder

1 can chopped tomatoes (15 oz.)

1 apple cider cup

1 medium sliced onion

1 tbsp olive oil extra-virgin 1 teaspoon cayenne pepper

(fifteen-ounce cans) white navy beans, cleaned and drained teaspoon sea salt 2 bay leaves 2 tblsp garlic powder 2 cups Bone broth from chickens or store-bought chicken broth

3 cups cooked chicken, chopped (see "Rotisserie" Chicken Basics) Black pepper, freshly ground

1 tblsp. cayenne

Directions:

Combine the chicken, beans, onion, tomatoes, broth, cider, bay leaves, olive oil, garlic powder, chili powder, salt, cumin, cinnamon, and cayenne pepper in a slow cooker. Season with black pepper.

Set your cooker's lid to low and lock it in place. Allow for an eight-hour cooking time.

Remove the bay leaves and toss them out. Before serving, stir in the apple cider vinegar until well combined.

Information about the calories: calorie count: 469 8 grams total fat 46 g total carbohydrate, 13 g sugar, 9 g fiber, 51 g protein Sodium: 1,047 milligrams

CHICKEN WITH VEGETABLES IN THE WINTER

Preparation time: 5 min Cooking Time: 30 min Servings Count 2\sIngredients:

1 leaf of bay

1 grated carrot

1 pound chicken breasts, chopped 1 turnip, chopped cups chicken stock 1 cup green beans, diced 1 onion, chopped 1 parsnip, chopped

2 quarts whipped cream olive oil, 2 tbsp.

2 tsp chopped fresh thyme To taste, season with salt and pepper.

Directions:

Warm the olive oil in a pan over medium heat. After three minutes of sautéing the onion, add the stock, carrot, turnip, parsnip, chicken, and bay leaf. Bring to a boil, then reduce to a low heat for approximately 20 minutes.

Cook for seven minutes after adding the asparagus. To serve, discard the bay leaf, stir in the whipped cream, adjust the salt, and top with fresh thyme. Information about the calories: 483 calories 32.5g fat (net) Carbohydrates: 6.9 g 33 g protein

BEET HUMMUS HUMMUS HUMMUS HUMMUS

Preparation time: 5 min 0 minutes to prepare Servings Count 2\sIngredients:

14 teaspoon chili powder

12 cup extra virgin olive oil

12 teaspoon oregano

12 teaspoon salt

12 teaspoon cumin

a third of a cup of chickpeas a single garlic clove

1 fresh ginger nub 1 roasted beet (skinless) 1 tsp curry powder

1 tbsp maple syrup

sunflower seeds (tbsp.) One lemon's juice

Instructions: In a food processor, combine all of the ingredients until smooth, then garnish with sunflower seeds.

Enjoy!

Information about the calories: 423 calories per serving; 13.98 grams of protein; 24.26 grams of fat 40.13 g carbohydrates

STIR FRY BROCCOLI AND BLACK BEANS

fifteen minutes to prepare Cooking time: fifteen minutes Servings Count 4 ingredients: 1 tablespoon sesame oil garlic cloves, finely chopped 2 cups black beans, cooked

2 tablespoons finely chopped ginger Broccoli florets, 4 cups

sesame seeds, 4 tblsp. a generous teaspoon of red chili flakes turmeric powder, a pinch

to flavor lime juice (not necessary) To taste, season with salt Pour enough water into the large frying pan to cover the bottom by an inch. On the deep frying pan, place a strainer.

Broccoli florets should be placed in the strainer. Broccoli should be steamed for around six minutes.

Preheat a large frying pan over medium heat. Pour sesame oil into the pan. Add sesame seeds, chili flakes, ginger, garlic, turmeric powder, and salt to the hot oil. Sauté for 2 minutes, or until fragrant.

Sauté the steamed broccoli and black beans until they are well cooked.

Stir in the lime juice.

Warm it up and serve.

Information about the calories: 196 calories per serving; 11.2 grams of protein; 7.25 grams of fat 23.45 g carbohydrate

ONIONS AND CARAMELIZED PEARS

Preparation time: 5 min Cooking Time: 35 min Servings Count 4 Ingredients: 1 tablespoon extra virgin olive oil

hard red pears, quartered and cored 2 red onions, peeled and sliced into wedges

Season with salt and pepper to taste.

Preheat the oven to 425 degrees Fahrenheit.

Sprinkle olive oil over the pears and onion on a baking dish.

Season to taste with salt and pepper.

Bake for a little more than half an hour in your oven.

Enjoy your meal!

Calories: 101; Fat: 4g; Carbohydrates: 0; Protein: 0; Carbohydrates: 0; Carbohydrates: 0; 17 g Carbohydrates 1 gram of protein

MASH OF CAULIFLOWER AND BROCCOLI

Preparation time: 5 min Cooking Time: 10 min Servings Count 6 Ingredients: 1 large cauliflower head, sliced into bits 1 floret of broccoli from a small head 1 tsp sodium

3 tbsp olive oil (extra virgin) salt and pepper to taste

Directions:

Put some oil in a saucepan and heat it up.

Place the cauliflower and broccoli in the pot.

To taste, season with salt and pepper.

Continue stirring until the vegetables are tender.

If necessary, add water.

Use a food processor or a potato masher to purée the veggies after they've been cooked.

Enjoy your meal!

Information about the calories: calorie count: 39 3 g of fat 2 g Carbohydrates 0.89 g protein

PLATTER WITH CILANTRO AND AVOCADO

fifteen minutes to prepare 0 minutes to prepare Servings Count 6 ingredients: 14 cup chopped fresh cilantro 12 lime juice

1 large ripe tomato, chopped green bell pepper, chopped 1 sweet onion, peeled, pitted, and diced avocados Season with salt and pepper as needed.

Place the onion, bell pepper, tomato, avocados, lime, and cilantro in a medium-sized container.

Toss everything together well.

Depending on your preference, season with salt and pepper.

Enjoy your meal!

Information about the calories: Calories: 126 Fat grams: 10 10 g Carbohydrates 2 g protien

COUSCOUS CITRUS WITH HERBS

Preparation time: 5 min Cooking time: fifteen minutes Servings Count 2\sIngredients:

12 teaspoon butter 14 cup water 14 orange, diced

1 teaspoon spices (Italian) a third of a cup of couscous

a third teaspoon of salt

a quarter-cup of orange juice

Fill the pan halfway with water and orange juice.

Combine the orange, Italian seasoning, and salt in a mixing bowl.

Bring the liquid to a boil, then remove from the heat.

Add the butter and couscous to the pan. Close the cover after fully stirring.

Allow 10 minutes for the couscous to rest.

Information about the calories: 149 calories Carbs: 28.5 Carbs: 1.9 Fat: 1.9 Fiber: 2.1 Fat: 1.9 Fat: 1.9 Fat: 1.9 Fat: 1.9 Fat: 1.9 Fat: 1.9 Fat: 4.1 g protein

BEANS WITH SPINACH AND GARBANZO

Preparation time: 5–10 minutes

Cooking time: 0 minutes Servings Count 4 items:

12 onion (diced)

1 tablespoon olive oil 12 teaspoon cumin

12 ounces garbanzo beans 10 ounces spinach, diced

Fill a frying pan halfway with olive oil and set aside.

Set the temperature to medium to low.

Cook for five minutes after adding the onions and garbanzo beans.

Cumin, garbanzo beans, spinach, and sunflower seeds are added to the mix.

Gently crush with a spoon.

Cook with care.

Enjoy your meal!

Information about the calories: calorie count: 90 4 g of fat 11 g carbohydrate, 4 g protein

SALAD WITH COUSCOUS

fifteen minutes to prepare Cooking time: six minutes Servings Count 4\sIngredients:

14 teaspoon black pepper, ground

34 teaspoon coriander powder

12 tsp sodium

a quarter teaspoon of paprika

a quarter teaspoon of turmeric 1 tablespoon unsalted butter

2 oz. canned chickpeas, drained 1 cup chopped fresh arugula

2 oz. chopped sun-dried tomatoes 1 oz. crumbled Feta cheese

1 tblsp. rapeseed oil a third of a cup of couscous

1/3 cup stock made from chicken

Prepare the chicken stock by bringing it to a boil.

Combine the couscous, black pepper, ground coriander, salt, paprika, and turmeric in a mixing bowl. Add the chickpeas and the butter. Close the cover after thoroughly mixing the ingredients.

Allow six minutes for the couscous to soak in the heated chicken broth.

Meanwhile, combine arugula, sun-dried tomatoes, and Feta cheese in a mixing container.

Combine the cooked couscous and canola oil in a mixing bowl.

Toss the salad well.

Information about the calories: calorie count: 18 calorie count: 18 calorie count: 18 calorie count: 9 % fat Carbs: 21.1 Fiber: 3.6 Fiber: 3.6 Fiber: 3.6 Fiber: 3.6 Fiber: 3.6 Fiber: 3.6 Fiber: 3.6 Fiber 6 g protein

POLENTA CREAMY

Preparation time: 8 minutes Cooking Time: 45 min Servings Count 4\sIngredients:

12 cup heavy cream 12 cup of water 1 polenta cup

1/3 cup grated Parmesan 2 cups stock (chicken)

Place the polenta in a saucepan and bring to a boil.

In a large mixing bowl, combine the water, chicken stock, cream, and Parmesan cheese. Mix the polenta well.

Preheat the oven to 355 degrees Fahrenheit.

Preheat the oven to 350°F and bake the polenta for 45 minutes.

Before serving, carefully stir together the prepared food with the spoon.

Calories: 208; Fat: 5.3; Fiber: 1; Carbs: 32.2; Protein: 8; Calories: 208; Fat: 5.3; Fiber: 1; Carbs: 32.2; Protein: 8 CRISPY CORN

Preparation time: 8 minutes Cooking Time: 5 min Servings Count 3\sIngredients:

12 teaspoon paprika powder

12 tblsp salt 34 tblsp chili powder 1 cup kernels of corn

1 tablespoon flour (coconut) 1 teaspoon of water

a third of a cup of canola oil

Instructions: Combine corn kernels, salt, and coconut flour in a mixing container.

Pour in the water and stir in the corn with a spoon.

Heat up the canola oil in the frying pan.

Place the corn kernels mixture in the oven and cook for four minutes. It should be stirred every now and again.

When the corn kernels are crispy, transfer them to the dish and dry them with a paper towel.

Add the chili pepper and paprika powder. Mix everything up well.

Information about the calories: 179 calories, fifteen grams of fat Carbs: 11.3 g Fiber: 2.4 g Fiber: 2.4 g Fiber: 2.4 g Fiber: 2.4 g Fiber: 2.1 CUCUMBER YOGURT SALAD WITH MINT PROTEIN

fifteen minutes to prepare 0 minutes to prepare Servings Count 2\sIngredients:

14 cup coconut milk (organic)

14 cup mint leaves (organic)

14 teaspoon Himalayan pink salt

12 cup organic red onion, chopped 1 tbsp extra virgin olive oil 1 tbsp organic plain goat yogurt 1 tablespoon fresh organic lime juice 1 teaspoon organic dill weed sliced organic cucumbers

Cut the red onion, dill, cucumbers, and mint into small pieces and combine them in a large container.

Blend until they're completely smooth.

Toss the cucumber salad with the dressing and combine well. Serve after chilling for at least 1 hour.

Enjoy!

Calories: 207 kcal Protein: 6.9 g Fat: 13.87 g Carbohydrates: 18.04 g Nutritional Information: Calories: 207 kcal Protein: 6.9 g Fat: 13.87 g Carbohydrates: 18.04 g

RICE WITH WHEATBERRY CURRY

fifteen minutes to prepare

Cooking time: 1 hour 15 minutes

Servings Count 5\sIngredients:

14 cup of milk

rice (12 cup)

wheat berries (1 cup)

1 teaspoon curry powder 1 tsp sodium

4 tablespoons extra virgin olive oil 6 cups stock (chicken) In a skillet, combine the wheatberries and chicken stock.

Cook the mixture for an hour over medium heat with the lid closed.

After that, add the rice, olive oil, and salt.

Completely combine all ingredients.

Combine the milk and curry paste in a mixing bowl.

In the rice-wheatberry combination, pour in the curry liquid and stir well.

Cook the food for 15 minutes with the lid closed.

When the rice is done, the rest of the dinner is ready.

Information about the calories: 232 cals 15 pounds of fat Carbohydrates: 23.5 Fiber: 1.4 Protein: 3.9

SALAD WITH FARRO AND ARUGULA

fifteen minutes to prepare Cooking Time: 35 min Servings Count 2\sIngredients:

12 c. farro

12 tsp black pepper, freshly ground

12 teaspoon seasoning (Italian)

12 teaspoon extra virgin olive oil

12 cup stock (chicken) 1 tbsp lemon juice 1 cucumber, diced 1 teaspoon salt 1 cup chopped arugula

Directions: Combine farro, salt, and chicken stock in a skillet and stir to combine.

Boil for a little more than half an hour with the lid closed.

Meanwhile, combine the other ingredients in the salad container.

Bring the farro to room temperature before adding it to the salad container.

Toss the salad well.

Calories 92 Calories 92 Calories 92 Calories 92 Calories 92 Calories 2.3 g of fat, 2 g of fiber Carbohydrates: 15.6 FETA: 3.9 protein SALAD WITH CHEESE

fifteen minutes to prepare 0 minutes to prepare Servings Count 2 Ingredients: 1 tablespoon olive oil (extra virgin) cucumbers, 1 teaspoon balsamic vinegar

feta cheese, 30 g 4 green onions

4 tomatillos

Salt

Cucumbers and tomatoes should be chopped into cubes.

Onions should be sliced thinly.

Feta cheese should be crushed.

Tomatoes, onions, and cucumbers should all be mixed together.

Combine the olive oil, vinegar, and a pinch of salt in a small mixing bowl.

feta cheese should be added.

Have fun eating!

Calories: 221 kcal Protein: 9.24 g Fat: 13.84 g Carbohydrates: 17.18 g Nutritional Information: Calories: 221 kcal Protein: 9.24 g Fat: 13.84 g

STRAWBERRY SALSA WITH FRESH STRAWBERRY

fifteen minutes to prepare 0 minutes to prepare Yield: 6–8 people

Ingredients:

14 c. lime juice, freshly squeezed

12 cup cilantro, chopped

12 cup coarsely chopped red onion 12 teaspoon grated lime zest 1-2 deseeded jalapeos 2 pounds fresh ripe strawberries, hulled and diced 2 kiwis, peeled and chopped 2 tsp. honey (raw)

In a large mixing bowl, whisk together lime juice, lime zest, and honey.

Add the rest of the ingredients and stir well. Cover and leave aside for a few minutes to allow the flavors to meld.

Calories: 119 kcal Protein: 9.26 g Fat: 4.38 g Carbohydrates: 11.73 g Nutritional Information: Calories: 119 kcal Protein: 9.26 g Fat: 4.38 g

CPSIA information can be obtained
at www.ICGtesting.com
Printed in the USA
LVHW060751040422
715224LV00006B/108